HEALTHY KNEES TOTAL KNEE REPLACEMENT

The 5 Pillar Plan to Prepare for Surgery and
Get the Most Out of Your New Knee

HEALTHY KNEES TOTAL KNEE REPLACEMENT

The 5 Pillar Plan to Prepare for Surgery and Get the Most Out of Your New Knee

ROBIN ROBERTSON
WITH CONTRIBUTOR DR. STEPHEN BLACK

Niche Pressworks
INDIANAPOLIS, IN

DEDICATION

Healthy Knees Total Knee Replacement is dedicated to my husband, Doug Robertson, for nursing me through my many knee surgeries, giving me the "elevator arm" when I couldn't step down the stairs on my own, for comforting and counseling me when difficult decisions arose, for always being there as my best friend and cheerleader along my long and painful knee journey. With my two new knees, I hope that we have many knee-pain-free adventures for years to come.

ACKNOWLEDGMENTS

Thank you to Dr. Stephen Black for his contribution in this book in the section called "Eat Smarter: Prepare for and Recover from Surgery Faster with the Right Nutrition." What you eat is not often talked about as a part of your surgery preparation and recovery. I wish I had known this information many surgeries ago and am grateful for his contribution so you can take advantage of his advice now.

TABLE OF CONTENTS

IF YOU WANT THE VERY BEST OUTCOME WITH YOUR TOTAL KNEE REPLACEMENT, THIS BOOK IS FOR YOU

Making the decision to replace your knee is big and life-changing.

This short book will help you prepare for your knee surgery so you go in stronger, recover faster, and ultimately become the strongest you can be with your new knee.

The weaker you are before your surgery, the weaker you will be after. When you are weak, it makes full recovery harder. Conversely, the stronger you are before going under the knife, the stronger you'll be to start your recovery. Wouldn't you like to start out stronger?

MY LIFETIME WITH KNEE ISSUES IS YOUR SHORTCUT TO GREAT KNEE OUTCOMES

Hi, my name is Robin Robertson, and I've had multiple knee surgeries of my own (you'll read my story in Chapter 4), I've learned a lot about the right ways (and wrong ways) to prepare for and recover from surgeries. Even with knee surgeries, I've maintained a healthy, active life and want to share with you the secrets to strong knees that will carry you far.

I am passionate about helping you have your own healthy knees, and I write to you from a very practical background of trial and error, along with training, research, and application. I own the Bellingham Training and Tennis Club, am a certified personal trainer and USA Cycling Coach. I have merged my own life experiences with these practical applications to bring you this book and two others: *Healthy Knees Strength* and *Healthy Knees Cycling*. Since 2015 my team and I have used our Club as a "test kitchen" for our Healthy Knees programs and have seen amazing results from hundreds of clients in our Healthy Knees programs. The Healthy Knees Formula online program (www.healthykneesformula.com) gives additional guidance at the next level up from what this book has to offer.

This book is for you if you are considering knee replacement (or any knee surgery for that matter), have scheduled surgery, or are already done with knee surgery and want better results. We work with many clients who come in suffering from knee pain (some with and some without knee replacements) and leave feeling stronger, invigorated, and confident in their knee movement.

In this book, I describe the 5 Pillar Plan to improve strength before your surgery, as well as the activities you can continue with after surgery and completing your physical therapy. These supplemental activities and new habits will help you get better results in the long run. And that is what your surgery is about: to get your knees working great again and give you back the activities you love in life.

As a part of this plan, I'm sharing very important information about pre- and post-surgery nutrition from Dr. Stephen Black. His perspective opens an often-ignored channel to prepare better for and recover faster from surgery.

Yes, it takes work, and YES! You can do this! What you do before and after surgery matters. It takes consistent work to get great results, but it's not hard or onerous. Don't worry; we'll help you every step of the way.

Wouldn't you like to feel like your knees are ready for anything? I want to help you feel great, whether it is walking downstairs without pain, getting out of a chair without help, or having the confidence to say YES to a fun adventure, no matter how big or small.

I hope you will join me on this journey of making the best out of your knees so that you can have the knee strength and confidence to enjoy life.

CHAPTER 1

ADDRESSING THE DISTRESS: MAKING THE TOTAL KNEE REPLACEMENT DECISION

You either make a decision or a circumstance
makes a decision for you.
—ANONYMOUS

Does This Spiral of Pain Sound Familiar?

- Your knee hurts, and so you do less
- You are afraid to move and make it worse
- As you do less, you gain weight
- As you gain weight, moving hurts more
- And since it hurts more, you move even less
- And you gain more weight
- And your knees hurt more
- And you do even less

I was told when I was 24 years old that I had so much arthritis that I should have my knee replaced, but I was way too young for any doctor to do it, or any replacement parts to last "long enough." I spent the next 34 years doing everything I could to not have my knee replaced. Then, finally, came the time when the pain was overtaking my life, my activities were vastly reduced, and my knee was not functioning well.

I cried. I denied. I wrestled with all of the "what ifs" that come with major reconstructive surgery. Maybe you are feeling this same way.

Once you have a total knee replacement (TKR), there is no going back. The decision to replace your knee(s) is no small thing. The recovery is long, slow, and painful. It is a traumatic surgery! Skilled surgeons look more like diabolical carpenters as they carve away the ends of your bones to create the surface for the replacement implants. Sometimes it's better NOT to think about what really happens during surgery.

Should you or should you not replace your knee? You and your doctor are the only ones who can make that decision. If you are considering your options to reduce your knee pain, please seek guidance from your doctor. It's not a bad idea to get a second opinion as well. In Chapter 2, we'll cover some questions you can ask the doctors, but first, you have to explore the decision for yourself.

THE DECISION—IS YOUR QUALITY OF LIFE GOING DOWNHILL?
The decision to replace your knee becomes plainer as your quality of life diminishes.

Does It Hurt Bad Enough?

- Pain is always a motivator to make a change. Chronic pain can wear you down and lead to fatigue. It's like you have on the "pain cloak" and just have to get through the day.

- Different people have different pain tolerances for sure—but when enough is enough, you know it.

- Perhaps it is as simple as not being able to walk the errands that you used to do and having to sit out of other important routine activities.

- Or maybe you are taking a boatload of NSAIDs (non-steroidal anti-inflammatory drugs such as ibuprofen) to combat the pain and might be worried about the effects on your kidneys or stomach.

- Or one by one, the sports you enjoyed become more painful than they were fun. So you stop: stop skiing, stop running, stop hiking.

- Maybe your knee pain wakes you up in the middle of the night, and you are losing sleep. That can wreck a day...or more.

- Pain tolerance...how much can you/should you bear? It is not a badge of honor. Pain is exhausting. You shouldn't have to live in pain all of the time. Your own pain level will be the driver for when you talk with your doctor about options for your knee.

ARE YOUR MOVEMENTS LIMITED?

Losing functionality in your knee is another huge motivator for knee replacement. What is normal knee range of motion? The measurement expectations diminish with age and vary by sex, as shown in the Normal Joint Range of Motion Study.[1] This study states that knee flexion range of motion for females aged 45-69 is an average of 138 degrees, and for males is an average of 133 degrees. Are you losing functionality in your knee?

• If you can't fully straighten your knee, this will likely affect your walking gait, and you might start to have hip or low back trouble.

• If you can't fully bend your knee, this will have implications with functional movements, such as being able to squat or get on and off the floor.

• If you are a bicycle rider, you'll need 110 degrees bend in your knees in order to pedal. I'm pretty sure bicycling helped me keep at least that much range of motion for so many years of advanced arthritis. Before I had my first knee replacement, I was having trouble stepping over things and would sometimes awkwardly catch my foot because my knee wasn't bending enough.

---

1 Centers for Disease Control and Prevention, 2019. "Normal Joint Range of Motion Study." Accessed January 17, 2020. https://www.cdc.gov/ncbddd/jointrom/index.html

- Or perhaps osteoarthritis (degenerative joint disease) has set in, and you are advancing toward, or are already at, that "bone on bone" stage where the cartilage is no longer doing its job to protect your bones. Or maybe the osteoarthritis is producing bone spurs that are getting in the way of the mechanical movement in your knee.

If you are losing functionality in your knee, surgery may be an inevitable necessity, not just an option.

THE TRAUMA OF SURGERY

Total knee replacement is an invasive procedure that takes time for recovery. Be sure to consult with your doctor about the expectation for assistance at home post-surgery. Ask if you will be hospitalized or have out-patient surgery. Everyone comes into a TKR with different circumstances that may lead to different kinds of protocols. There are plenty of articles, blogs, and chat groups online that will give you different perspectives on how different people's surgeries turned out.

Physical Pain

You might be worried about how much it's going to hurt. I know I was! That is totally understandable and hard to predict. Different people react and respond differently to injury pain, neural response, and medication effectiveness.

Emotional Exhaustion

Pain is draining. If you've been living with pain for some time, you might just be at the point that you can't carry that burden any longer.

What If I'm Worse Off?

This was the question that haunted me prior to deciding to go ahead with the TKR. My knee was bad, but was it really that bad? I had that conversation with myself and my husband a hundred times.

There comes a time when you feel like it's the only choice to move forward with any hope that it will get better. Thankfully, both my knee replacements have been a blessing (after the recovery), and I wish that for you too. Luckily, you can control the outcomes to some extent!

Significant Recovery Time

How long it takes to recover and return to "normal" life varies and will depend, in part, on the preparation you do prior to surgery.

Everyone is Different

How fast and how well you recover depends a lot on where you are starting from. That's really why I wrote this book: to help you get to a better starting line. You'll typically start moving the day after surgery using a walker or crutches. Remember, this is a marathon, not a sprint. Take the long view and consider that you'll be 80% recovered in one year and 100% in two years. The more you work at it, the better you will be.

Physical Therapy (PT)

Some sort of PT typically starts right away, often before you even leave the hospital. It will be up to you, your doctor's advice, and your therapist regarding how many times per week and the number of weeks you'll work together. It will also depend on your diligence in doing the exercises, tolerance by your new knee, recovery rate, and probably what is allowed by your insurance.

Having Post-Surgery Help

You'll definitely want help at home for the first while after your surgery. Having someone to help provide meals, give assistance in getting dressed, bring ice bags for your knee, fluff your pillows, and help you be less miserable is soothing. How long you'll want help will depend on many factors that you can discuss with your doctor.

THE EXPENSE OF KNEE SURGERY

You may be worried about how much this knee is going to cost, not only in money outlay but also missed time at work. The average hospital charge for a knee replacement surgery is approximately $49,500[2], with an average hospital stay of 2.3 days. Partial knee replacements are typically 10-20 percent less because of the shorter hospital stay. Some people qualify for an "outpatient" TKR where you are sent home within 24 hours of the surgery. The average cost for outpatient TKR surgery may be 40 percent less.[3]

Insurance

You'll need your insurance to approve your surgery before moving ahead. Make sure you understand what they will and won't pay for.

I chuckled when I got my notice of approval for my right total knee replacement. Good thing I ended up with the correct body part!

---

2 Healthline. "Understanding Knee Replacement Costs: What's on the Bill?" Accessed February 11, 2020. https://www.healthline.com/health/total-knee-replacement-surgery/understanding-costs#1

3 "Becker's ASC Review, 2019. "Outpatient Joint Replacements at ASCS Cost 40% Less Than Hospital-Based Surgery: 3 Study Details"

Dear Patient:

The request for coverage of the service below is approved.

Specialty: ORTHOPEDICS

Service: L8699 Replacement body part

Start date: 11/12/19

Custom vs. "Off-the-Shelf," and Why It Matters

We all have the same construction of our knee joint: the thigh bone (femur) meets the lower leg bone (tibia), with the kneecap (patella) on top. But the shape of these bones can vary quite a bit.

There is a difference between genuine custom knees and "off the shelf" replacements. As my doctor had told me, for most people, the "off the shelf" knee works just fine as it comes in many different sizes. An important part of what your surgeon will do is to predict the size of your knee implant parts so that several options are available during surgery.

Correct component sizes facilitate proper knee motion after replacement and may decrease pain and need for revision.[4] Components that are too large may result in overhang and may irritate surrounding soft tissue, which reduces motion and doubles the odds of post-operative pain[5]. An off-the-shelf knee replacement is not necessarily the same shape as your natural bones.

---

4 Archives of Bone and Joint Surgery, 2018. "Total Knee Replacement Sizing: Shoe Size Is a Better Predictor for Implant Size than Body Height." Accessed January 18, 2020. https://www.ncbi.nlm.nih.gov/pmc/articles/PMC5867352/

5 Journal of Bone and Joint Surgery, 2010. "Overhang of the Femoral Component In Total Knee Arthroplasty: Risk Factors And Clinical Consequences." Accessed January 18, 2020. https://www.ncbi.nlm.nih.gov/pubmed/20439656

Custom knees, on the other hand, are designed specifically for the unique dimensions of each individual's bones. Whether or not your insurance will cover a custom knee is another story and likely will have to do with how your surgeon codes it for insurance request. Not all surgeons work with custom knees but be sure to inquire about this option.

I had custom knees for both of my replacements and am very happy with the results. I cannot speak to the process by which all custom knees are created, but for mine, it started with a CT scan 6-weeks prior to the surgery date. That gave the specific dimensions of my knee for the company (Conformis) to create my knee replacement parts.

I even asked to meet my knee just before my surgery, and my surgeon was kind enough to indulge me. Don't worry; it was still sterile inside its shipping box.

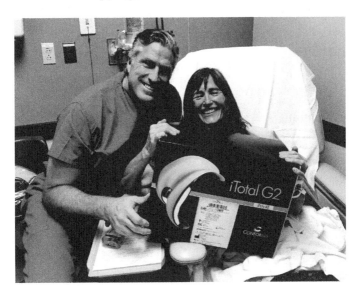

THE HOPE THAT A NEW KNEE BRINGS

We all have the HOPE that a knee joint replacement will take away the pain and give us back mobility. But the replacement itself can only give us a knee that functionally works. The key to success is having strong muscles that support your knee's actions, and that is exactly what we get to later in this book.

The winning combination is New Knee + The Right Exercises + Good Nutrition = Best Results. The right kind of exercise is KEY because the wrong kind can ultimately reduce the life of the joint.

WHAT YOU SHOULD AND SHOULDN'T DO WITH A TKR

Low and no-impact exercises are recommended for total knee replacements. But what does that mean for the knee?

"Impact" refers to the force that goes through the knee joint caused by your foot striking the ground. As you walk, run, or jump, the forces transmitted are multiplied by your body weight:

> » Walking 2-3 X body weight [6]
> » Jogging 4-5 X body weight
> » Running 6-14 X body weight[7]
> » Jumping 9-10+ X body weight

There are also shear forces through the knee caused by gravity and resistance (like when you slow down or come to a sudden stop).

---

6 PMC US national Library of Medicine, National Institutes of Health. (2013). Knee Joint Forces: Prediction, Measurement, and Significance. Retrieved on 12/6/19 from https://www.ncbi.nlm.nih.gov/pmc/articles/PMC3324308/

7 Medscape.com (2015) Joint Loading in Runners Does Not Initiate Knee Osteoarthritis. Retrieved on 12/6/19 from: http://www.azisks.com/wp-content/uploads/2017/04/Joint-Loading-in-Runners-Does-Not-Initiate-Knee-Osteoarthritis.pdf

Before your knee replacement, you may feel pain from how your knee is moving with these shear forces when walking up or down a hill, up or down a flight of stairs. Your new knee is designed to be stable and handle this.

Low- or no-impact activities recommended by most surgeons include[8] walking, swimming, golf, driving, light hiking, biking, ballroom dancing, and other low-impact sports. Activities recommended to avoid for the rest of your life include running, jogging, jumping, or other high-impact sports.

HOW LONG DOES YOUR NEW KNEE LAST? THE FACTORS THAT CONTRIBUTE

A quick internet search reveals articles that agree with estimates my doctor made—longevity of 20-25 years for a total knee replacement if you take care of it. That means keeping a healthy weight and staying away from impact sports and a lot of lateral movement.

Parts Fail

Long-term failure may occur because the bond between the bone and implant has loosened over time, or a part of the implant (typically the replacement meniscus) has worn down.[9]

Your Weight

Your body weight makes a big difference to the wear and tear in both your old knees and your new one. If you reference the

---

8 OrthoInfo from the American Academy of Orthopaedic Surgeons, 2015. "Total Knee Replacement." Accessed January 18, 2020. https://orthoinfo.aaos.org/en/treatment/total-knee-replacement/

9 Cleveland Clinic, 2019. "How long Does a Hip or Knee Replacement Last?" Accessed January 18, 2020. https://health.clevelandclinic.org/how-long-does-a-hip-or-knee-replacement-last/

information above about impact forces, you'll quickly see how carrying an extra 10 pounds, 50 pounds, or, really, any excess weight will affect your knee.

Think about this; when walking, there is 2-3 times your body weight in force through your knee. An extra 20 pounds add up to 40-60 additional pounds of force in your knee just while walking. The more you weigh, the bigger the forces. Excessive force in the knee can add up to one of the reasons that knee joints fail.

Protecting your knees through maintaining a healthy weight is one of the very best things you can do.

YOUR ACTIVITY

What you do (or don't do) with your new knee may play a significant role in how long it lasts. The activities recommended for total knee replacements include no-impact and low-impact movement. If you choose otherwise—and I know plenty of people with knee replacements who do things like play tennis or downhill ski—the tradeoff may be that you are reducing the "lifespan" of your knee replacements, but enjoying life's activities that you love. That is a decision that only you can make.

I bet you'll want your new knees to last as long as possible and prolong the risk of a "revision" surgery, which is a replacement of your replacement. If that's the case, I advise you to stick to the recommended activities in order to protect your knees.

That may mean that you are letting go of some of your favorites (mine were running and skiing the moguls), and this can feel quite traumatic. I was a collegiate runner. My life revolved around running and studying and working. A big part of who I was had to change because of the outrageous amount of arthritis I already had. It was definitely a mind shift that I could and should do something different and better for my knees. It is a choice. You can choose a good attitude or have a poor one about the changes you need to make and see it as a new opportunity or a complete loss. I acknowledged how much I loved running and the joy that it gave me, but it became time for something new and different. I went forth with a positive attitude. I hope you, too, can make this positive mental shift.

There are so many fun things to do that are good for your knees. My very favorites are riding a bike and travel—and when you put the two together, it's a pretty awesome way to see the world. Get creative with the great ways to take care of you and your knees and still enjoy life!

AND THE "WHAT IFS"

One of the things everyone probably ponders for knee replacements is if it is going to work. This was the big showstopper for so many years for me—I was afraid. Afraid that it would not work, might cause more pain, might cause a post-surgical infection, would make me worry about blood clots (and worse), and ultimately, might have to be replaced again in 20-25 years, even if everything else went as well as it could.

Personally, the tradeoff was well worth it. I traded a chronically painful knee with a snap and a pop when I walked and cycled for a pain-free joint that has a hard "knock" when I walk. I'll take the pain-free knock any day. Like me, there is a reasonable chance that your knee will not feel completely "normal" afterward.[10] But that "what if" should not scare you away from relief.

There is definitely a LOT to worry about before a surgery. Take the time to discuss all of your concerns with your surgeon. Ultimately, you need to be comfortable enough to say yes to the risks to move ahead.

HOW TO MAKE THE BEST OF YOUR TKR?

To Sum It Up: Get Stronger and Stay Positive!

If you go into surgery weak, you come out weak. If you go into surgery strong with a higher level of fitness, it MAKES SENSE that you will exit surgery at a higher starting point than others who have not prepared. Research shows statistically significant improvements in all measures of outcome when patients participate in an exercise program prior to surgery.[11] Other studies show that your mental state going into surgery is also an important factor in your outcome [12]

---

10 Harvard Health Publishing, 2016. "Knee Replacement: Life Changing or a Disappointment?" Accessed January 22, 2020. https://www.health.harvard.edu/blog/knee-replacement-life-changing-disappointment-2016082410095

11 International Journal of Orthopaedic and Trauma Nursing, 2018. "Does Physiotherapy Prehabilitation Improve Pre-Surgical Outcomes and Influence Patient Expectations Prior To Knee and Hip Joint Arthroplasty?" Accessed January 11, 2020. https://www.sciencedirect.com/science/article/abs/pii/S1878124117301326

12 BioMed Research International, 2015. "What Augmented Physical Activity and Empowerment Can Bring to Patients Receiving Total Knee Replacement: Content, Implementation, and Comparative Effectiveness of a New Function-Tailored Care Pathway in a Routine Care Setting." Accessed January 11, 2020. https://www.hindawi.com/journals/bmri/2015/745864/abs/

One of my favorite sayings is "What you think is where you go"—kind of an adaptation of Henry Ford's "Whether you think you can, or you think you can't—you're right." Keeping a positive frame of mind, imagining the outcome you want, and working toward that outcome will make a difference.

I like to think of preparing for surgery as the same as preparing for an athletic event. If you are going to have surgery, go at it with all you've got so you will have the best chances for a great outcome.

An athlete trying to have the best outcome for their event needs to train in a way that supports their movements. A weightlifter will not lift more weight unless he/she does the work and trains for it. A swimmer will not go faster if they spend no time in the pool. A runner will not break a 6-minute mile if they aren't out running and training. A cyclist is not going to go longer or faster without putting in the miles.

If your knee and leg go into surgery weak, they are not going to magically come out stronger after the surgery. You will emerge with a new joint, but all the muscles that support the movement of the joint are the same (or worse because of the trauma).

If you go into surgery physically stronger, you will come out of surgery at a higher starting point than your friend who did nothing to prepare ahead of time. It is likely your recovery time will be shorter, and you'll feel better faster.

SUMMARY

Making the decision to have your knee replaced is no small thing. It is an invasive surgery that comes with physical pain and emotional drain as you work through recovery. It can, with good outcomes, change your life for the better. No more knee pain! To get the most out of your new knee, it is best to go into surgery as strong as possible and to continue to do the strength and movement training after physical therapy, so you will get stronger and able to do the things you love in life.

CHAPTER 2

SMART QUESTIONS TO ASK YOUR DOCTOR AS PART OF YOUR TKR DECISION

Here is a list of questions to ask your doctor as you consider a TKR. You should know the details of your procedure and the expectations for recovery. The questions are organized by category: Costs and Considerations, Replacement Information, Pre-Surgery, Surgery Procedure, and Post-Surgery

COSTS AND CONSIDERATIONS

- How much does a knee replacement cost?
- How do I find out if/how much my insurance will pay?
- Are there additional costs to consider? Will I need any special equipment? (e.g., a special chair for showering, ramp instead of stairs)
- Can I avoid surgery?
- Are there alternatives I should consider first? (injections of platelet-rich plasma or stem cell, for example)
- Do I have a choice over what hospital I go to, and does it make a difference in procedure or costs?

- Are there any risks in delaying the replacement of my knee?
- What are the potential complications?
- How can I prepare now for surgery later? (in addition to what you are learning in this book—wink-wink)
- Is there an option for a "minimally invasive " knee replacement surgery? (And what does that mean?)

REPLACEMENT INFORMATION
- How many years will my TKR last?
- Do you offer a "custom" knee replacement option or only an "off the shelf" option?
- Will I keep my PCL? (The posterior cruciate ligament (PCL) connects the femur to the tibia inside the knee joint toward the back of the knee. A PCL retaining implant will keep your PCL intact and remove less bone during the surgery.[13] A PCL substituting implant will remove your PCL. Discuss with your doctor the pros and cons of your options.)
- What should I expect for range of motion post-surgery? How far is my replacement rated to bend? (Not all knee replacement parts are alike. In general, you should expect to regain what you have currently and may exceed that with diligent work. My doctor said any TKR at 120 degrees or greater is an "A.")

13 Drugwatch. "Knee Replacement." Accessed March 1, 2020. https://www.drugwatch.com/knee-replacement/

- What happens to the kneecap? Is it resurfaced? All knee replacements have a part that attaches to the thigh bone (femur) and one that attaches to the shin bone (tibia). Some, but not all, have a component that is attached to the underside of the patella so that it glides smoothly against the femoral and tibial implants.
- Is the joint cemented in place, or does your doctor use a "cementless" technique where the bone grows into the implant?
- What is the knee replacement made of? Should I worry about biocompatibility or that it could corrode in my body? The different types of implants are categorized by the materials that rub together when you flex your knee.[14]

  » **Metal on Plastic:** Most common type with a metal femoral and tibial with a plastic (polyethylene) meniscus. Common metals include cobalt-chromium, titanium, zirconium, and nickel.

  » **Ceramic on Plastic:** Uses a ceramic (or ceramic-coated metal) femoral and tibial implant with a plastic meniscus. If you have a sensitivity to nickel, you might consider the ceramic option.

  » **Ceramic on Ceramic:** Does not include the plastic meniscus.

  » **Metal on Metal:** Does not include the plastic meniscus.

---

14 Harvard Health Publishing. "4 Types of Knee Implants." Accessed March 1, 2020. https://www.health.harvard.edu/pain/4-types-of-knee-implants

- Concerns about materials:
  - » Plastic parts may wear away tiny particles that can trigger an immune reaction, possibly causing bone to break down, leading to loosening and possible failure of the implant.
  - » Metal parts may wear (especially metal on metal implants), and traces of metal can cause inflammation, pain, and possible organ damage.
  - » Ceramic on ceramic may squeak when you walk and can shatter under heavy pressure, requiring surgery for removal.
  - » Any of the joints may "knock" when you walk as they are hard surfaces bearing the impact of every step.

PRE-SURGERY

- Do I need to stop taking medications before surgery?
- What do I need to do at home to prepare for post-surgery? For example, make sure you have a clear path from bed to bathroom to kitchen that can accommodate a walker or crutches.
- Is there a "joint class?" Some surgeons or hospitals offer a pre-surgery class that helps you to prepare for surgery with tips on how to prepare your home and what to expect.
- Should I learn to use crutches or a walker before surgery?
- Do I need to lose weight before surgery?
- Is there anything I can do pre-surgery to lower the risk of infection or complications?
- How much time should I plan to take off from work? This answer will vary based on the physical demands of your job.

- Before surgery, should I schedule my post-surgery, outpatient physical therapy sessions? Some therapists can be booked up for a long time. How many sessions per week will your doctor prescribe?

SURGERY PROCEDURE

- What is the surgical procedure?
- How long does the surgery take?
- Will staples, sutures, or glue be used to close the incision? Glue may result in more pleasing cosmetic results for a finer scar, while sutures and staples both puncture the skin, and staples generally leave a much wider scar than sutures or glue.
- What kind of anesthesia will be used? What are my options?
- How many days will I be in the hospital? Do I qualify for outpatient surgery (1 day at surgery center)?

POST-SURGERY

- Will I be in much pain post-surgery, and what are the options for medications?
- How soon before I start moving?
- Will I receive physical therapy in the hospital? At home?
- When will I start physical therapy at the therapist's office?
- Will I need a walker or crutches? Keep in mind that a walker puts most people into a forward-leaning anatomically incorrect position. Discuss with your doctor if you are a good candidate to go straight to crutches instead of using a walker.
- How much help will I need after surgery? You can count on needing assistance in the first 24 hours, if not longer.

- When will I start physical therapy?
- How long before I will return to normal activity?

The answers will give you a lot of insight into the procedure of a total knee replacement as well as set the appropriate expectations for going into the procedure. The other key elements for surgery preparation and post-rehab are all of the things we talk about in this book.

CHAPTER 3

THE REALITY OF TKR RECOVERY

I was a little shocked after my first Total Knee Replacement about how much it hurt and how long the recovery period felt. Remember this: TKR is a traumatic surgery. Your knee has been opened up, muscles and ligaments moved out of the way, and the ends of your bones are actually being cut off and capped with the implants. Your body needs time to heal, and this takes a lot of energy.

Be patient with yourself. Sleep when you need to sleep. Follow doctor's orders. If you try to rush the healing process, you'll likely have a setback. Your knee will let you know that you've pushed it too hard because it will swell and hurt more. Let your knee be the boss. But at the same time, you'll have to get comfortable with being uncomfortable. There will be a certain amount of pain with the exercises that you and your physical therapist will need to discuss. This should diminish naturally as you progress through the phases of healing, though everyone's recovery will be different.

POST-SURGERY PHASES OF HEALING[15]

Days 1-3 Haemostasis (Damage Control)
- Construction of blood vessels
- Aggregation of platelets to form clots
- Leukocytes to fight off infection

Days 4-7 Inflammation (Repair Begins, Then Continues)
- Use ice for swelling
- Collagen lays down the matrix for new tissue formation
- Waste management systems remove necrotic tissue and generally clear out junk

Day 20 Proliferation (Healing and Growth of New Tissue)
- Consider compression for swelling, mobilization starts, use lymphatic massage to help with fluid draining
- Increasing fibrinogen and collagen to provide structure
- Epidermal cells migrate
- Granulation tissue forms as the base for skin healing

21 Days to 2 Years: Closure and Remodeling
- Collagen continues to strengthen repair of the wound
- New tissues get stronger
- Bones heal

---

15 Medfit Conference, 2020. Presentation by Dr. Stephen Black.

BUT WHAT DOES IT FEEL LIKE?

Everyone's response to surgery is different, and I hope you sleep like a baby and have no pain post-op. However, here is what it was like for me:

> The first week was very difficult and painful. Sleep was like a rotisserie chicken: I would find a comfy spot for an hour or so, then wake up roll around, repeat. There were times I'd get ice bags and pack my knee just to cut the pain and fall asleep. I watched a lot of movies.

> My physical therapist recommended in the first part of recovery, especially the first two weeks, to focus on reducing swelling and improving range of motion, not on weight-bearing strength exercises. You may feel like you are in a fog and need a lot of sleep. You may need to take an NSAID (non-steroidal anti-inflammatory drugs like ibuprofen), and possibly narcotic pain meds as needed. I know a few folks who successfully completed recovery without using narcotics by focusing on good hydration, proper nutrition, and supplements.

> Three weeks after my first TKR, I returned to work half-time. It was four weeks for my 2nd knee, partly because it was over the holidays, partly because of the pain. You can probably drive again, as long as you are not taking narcotics. It may be up to six weeks before driving if your gas pedal leg was the surgery leg.

Week 4 is a return to more normal activities, and you are likely to still feel tired. Honor the trauma your body has been through and take that time to rest. Resting and sleeping are when your body can heal. Energy may be low, which is to be expected. Your body is working hard to heal from this very invasive surgery.

Weeks 5 and 6, you might be getting to the point where you don't think about your knee pain all of the time! The danger is that you might be to the point with your physical therapy where your knee is feeling good and working well. But don't settle for "good enough!" There is still more to gain.

Six Weeks seems to be that magic number for total knee replacement, but the reality is there is still a long way to go. Are you fully recovered? No. It might be tempting to do MORE, but there are two big reasons not to push it: pain and inflammation. Listen to your body and listen to your physical therapist. Even though you think you can do more, your knee will tell you if that is the right amount of work or not. Pain and swelling mean you've done too much.

At seven weeks, the significant pain from the surgery has passed, but the healing pain and threat of swelling linger.

Somewhere around the 8th week, I remember taking a step and having NO pain. No pain! That is the promised land, and I hope you will get there too. But it did not mean I was fully recovered yet. It is easy to over-do it when you start feeling so good. Be mindful to only add a little more each day and see how you feel the next. If you are hurting, then it was too much, too soon.

In the 9th week, I definitely experienced swelling and discouragement because I overdid it. Too much walking, too much cycling. My PT reminded me that my knee was the "boss." So, I returned to a focus on reducing swelling and increasing range of motion.

Around 10-12 weeks, you might be ready to start work on going down stairs, using your new knee. That seems to be the last of the significant hurdles of normal function. Strength gains will be important to support your movement.

At three to six months, you may start to feel like "you" again and that your new knee is normal. Instead of the boss, your knee is now your co-pilot, helping you to make good choices. Hopefully, you no longer have swelling, and you feel like you have finished recovery. Maybe that could be "good enough." This is where I encourage you to do more and go past "just good enough" so you can have the very best results for your body and your knee. To achieve change, it is important to train as much as necessary, not as much as possible. Former athletes may have a challenge with the latter part of that statement. Just because you *could* do it doesn't mean that you *should* do it just yet.

And over the 24 months post-op, your body is still healing and becoming the best it will be with your new knee. That is why it is so important to follow the 5 Pillars that you will learn about in Chapter 7. But before we get there, I want to share with you my story of how I was able to postpone total knee replacement for so many years while living a healthy active life, even with advanced arthritis. Maybe you can successfully postpone your TKR too!

CHAPTER 4

HOW SUCCESSFULLY DELAYING MY KNEE REPLACEMENT SURGERY FOR 30 YEARS HELPS YOU RIGHT NOW

"We will either find a way or make one."
—HANNIBAL (247-182 BC)

I'm almost embarrassed to say it: I've had a total of 12 knee surgeries. This adds up to more experience under the scalpel of a surgeon than I wish on anyone. The short story is that each of my knees required surgery to fix a congenital condition in my meniscus cartilage. It began when I was just 13 years old. All the other surgeries continued as damage control for joint function as my osteoarthritis intensified. My surgeries have culminated with replacements in 2017 and 2019. Even through all of this knee pain and multiple knee surgeries, I found a way to stay fit and active.

I believe I was given a crappy pair of knees so I could take my experiences and help you learn from my successes and avoid my mistakes. Even with these knees of mine, I've ridden my bike around the world (between surgeries number 4 and 5) and have started my bicycle journey across the USA (between surgeries 9 through 12). I want you, too, to feel ready and able to make your own adventures.

There were valuable lessons to be learned over the years. I've taken this experience and poured it into this book to help you with avoiding the pitfalls and directly reaching the triumphs.

Here Is What I Found to Give the Best Results:

- #1 Prepare for your surgery by getting stronger.
- #2 Diligently do the physical therapy post-surgery.
- #3 Continue with a strength training program. This is the key to long-term success.
- #4 Be consistent with riding a bike to keep your knees healthy.

Here was my biggest problem: my second surgery at 24 years old told me I needed to have my knee replaced because of the amount of osteoarthritis I already had.

Back then, in the 1980s, no doctor would consider a knee replacement for a patient that young because of the replacement joint's life span. It was known then that a single joint could be replaced two times, but three times? That was questionable. It has to do with making the boreholes in your joint bigger each time to secure the implant. Perhaps there will not be enough "bone space" for a third replacement. So, if I would have had my knee replaced at 24 years old and then replaced again, that would have gotten me to about age 60 at best with a big "what next" question mark. No one was willing to take that chance, especially me.

My doctor simply told me to quit all impact sports if I wanted to be able to walk when I was 30. I didn't get much more advice than that, and as a senior in college about to start my final track season, this was a life-changing blow. Not only did I have to quit competitive running at the collegiate level, but also, I began to worry about life ahead and *simply being able to walk.*

HOW I SPENT THE NEXT 30+ YEARS
TRYING NOT TO HAVE A KNEE REPLACEMENT

Since I planned to live to be 100 years old, I wanted to make sure my knees could get me there. WHEN to have your TKR is a question that is dictated by:

- Medical need
- Pain
- Disability or quality of life
- Timing and available help
- Insurance, or can I afford it?
- Your age

Doctors want you to be old enough to have knee replacement surgery. That qualifier has changed over time as the technology for knee replacements has improved, and they last longer. In the 1980s and '90s, the estimates were that 90% or more of knee or hip replacements would last 10-15 years[16]. My doctor suggested

---

16 Harvard health Publishing, 2018. "How Long Will My Hip or Knee Replacement Last?" Accessed January 22, 2020. https://www.health.harvard.edu/blog/how-long-will-my-hip-or-knee-replacement-last-2018071914272

20-25 years. A meta-analysis of the national joint replacement registry found that 82% of TKRs last 25 years.[17]

Really, at age 24 (in 1985) I just wanted to find a way to be active and cause no further damage to my knees. Swimming, riding a bike, and weight training became my go-to activities. I still had chronic joint pain that definitely flared up after I did something like a hiking in hilly terrain.

I vehemently did not want to have my knee replaced (for fear of the "what next") and tried everything possible to keep them strong. Cycling was good. Strength training was good. But those two activities weren't quite enough to overcome advancing arthritis. Over the years, I had injections of cortisone, hyaluronic acid, platelet-rich plasma, and even stem cells. Each bought me a little more time. I tried electro-stimulation, acupuncture, and massage to alleviate pain. I thought healing thoughts and visualized a strong and healthy knee. I did everything I could think of

Eventually, by 2017, the pain wore me down. My knee mechanics were failing, and it was time to make the ultimate decision to replace. My orthopedic surgeon had said if it weren't for riding a bike, lifting weights, and staying a healthy weight, I would have had to have my knee replaced at least ten years earlier. This knowledge and practice of what works (and doesn't work) is what I bring to this book for you.

---

17 The Lancet, 2019. "How Long Does a Knee Replacement Last? A Systematic Review and Meta-Analysis of Case Series and National Registry Reports with More Than 15 Years of Follow-Up." Accessed January 22, 2020. https://www.thelancet.com/journals/lancet/article/PIIS0140-6736(18)32531-5/fulltext

PAVING THE WAY FOR GREAT RESULTS
FOR YOUR NEW KNEES

We all have HOPE that the TKR surgery will bring a better result. What that hope also needs is action. That means training for the surgery like it is an athletic event and continuing post-rehab to strengthen your body to support your knees. AND IT WORKS! I followed this practice and was told I'm the "model patient" for success in joint replacement with a fast recovery and high function.

Two years later, I knew a lot more about what I was getting into, and my right knee was replaced with the same great results. I decided, for this knee, I didn't want to postpone as long as I could because I had plans for a big bike ride and wanted the surgery sooner so that I could get on with the recovery. Now is it your turn?

To start getting ready for your own TKR, it is helpful to understand a little more about how your knee works. We dive into that in our next chapter.

CHAPTER 5

HOW YOUR KNEE WORKS

WHY YOUR FEET, LEGS, HIPS, AND CORE ARE CRITICAL FOR YOUR KNEES

The Responsibility of Your Knee

Three bones come together to form your knee: your thigh bone (femur—the largest bone in your body), shin bone (tibia), and knee-cap (patella). Your knee is called a weight-bearing joint because when you stand, walk, skip, run, and jump, the forces of your body weight are going through the knee joint.

Your legs would be like walking on stilts if it wasn't for the hinge at your knee joint, allowing your legs to bend. Your knee is the largest and most complex of the joints that are made for free movement. It is not simply a hinge. As you bend and straighten your knee, the end of the thigh bone rolls against the top of the shin bone. There is some rotation of the shin bone as your leg straightens, known as the "screw home mechanism." In a TKR, the amount of rotational ability you keep and will depend on the type of implant whether or not you retain the posterior cruciate ligament. [18] [19] [20]

Your knee joint would not function very well if it were just the bones coming together because there would be too much friction. Instead, your knee is like a sealed compartment inside the joint capsule with synovial fluid to lubricate movement and nourish the cartilage. Synovial fluid is produced from a specialized layer of cells in the synovial lining on the inside of the knee's joint capsule.[21] There are actually two joints in the knee, with the kneecap (patellofemoral joint) separate from the thigh bone-shin bone articulated hinge (tibiofemoral joint). The meniscus cartilage acts like cushions between your thigh bone and shin bone. Articular cartilage is the "shrink-wrap" protection around the ends of your bones and underneath your kneecap, which also helps protect the bones from damage.

YOUR KNEE IS NOT JUST ABOUT THE KNEE

Your knee's health is affected by all of the body parts that work together to form movement from your feet to your back. This is called the kinetic chain. Let's start with the skeletal structure, our bones. Our bones are tied together at joints with ropes of dense connective tissue called ligaments. If it weren't for bones, we'd be a puddle on the floor.

---

18 Journal of Orthopedics, 2015. "Tibial Rotation Kinematics Subsequent To Knee Arthroplasty." Accessed Febrary 11, 2020. https://www.ncbi.nlm.nih.gov/pmc/articles/PMC4353994/

19 *Clinical Orthopaedics and Related Research*, 2008. "Changes in Knee Kinematics Reflect the Articular Geometry after Arthroplasty." Accessed February 11, 2020. https://www.ncbi.nlm.nih.gov/pmc/articles/PMC2584306/

20 Efort Open Reviews, 2018. "What Is a Balanced Knee Replacement?" Accessed February 11, 2020. https://online.boneandjoint.org.uk/doi/full/10.1302/2058-5241.3.180008

21 MDPI, 2015. "The Synovial Lining and Synovial Fluid Properties after Joint Athroplasty." Available as open access document. www.mdpi.com/journal/lubricants

Since we have structure, we need a way to move it. Our muscles are like pulleys that tug the bones in one direction or another at every joint. Our muscles are attached to bones with dense connective tissue called tendons. What happens at one joint can affect the other joints along the kinetic chain. When any of your muscles along this kinetic chain is weak, it will affect the joint movements, which can result in pain. Weakness in one or more muscles can cause compensations in another. What may have started with knee pain, stemming from another muscle weakness, may then be compounded by hip pain as your body compensates for the weakness.

LET'S START AT YOUR FEET AND WORK OUR WAY UP.

Your Feet Are Your Foundation

Your feet are your foundation, and troubles with your feet can cause knee pain. Your foot is crazy complicated with 26 bones, 33 joints, and more than 100 muscles, tendons, and ligaments[22]. Many of the muscles that control movement in the foot originate in your lower leg. If your feet roll in or out too far, this affects the ankle and alignment of the bones of the shin (tibia and fibula).

An easy way to see if your foot rolls one way or the other is to check the wear in your shoes. If you see one side of the heel more worn than the other, then you can guess that there may be foot alignment issues. Check with your doctor or see a podiatrist to investigate solutions.

---

22 Arthritis Foundation Anatomy of the Foot. Accessed January 4, 2020. https://www.arthritis.org/about-arthritis/where-it-hurts/foot-heel-and-toe-pain/foot-anatomy.php

If you've noticed uneven wear in your shoes before surgery, after your TKR you will want to replace them. (My husband would say I'm making this up just because I want new shoes. But I'm not, and it's true!) Your knee alignment may have changed, and that will put different stresses on your feet. What you don't want is an old pair of shoes pushing your foot into an old pattern of movement.

Your Lower Leg Controls Your Ankle, Foot, and Toes

Your lower leg is made up of two bones: the tibia (shin bone) and fibula (the smaller of the two bones). When you reach down to touch the front of your shin bone, that is your tibia; when you touch the outer side of your ankle, that is the end of the fibula. The muscles of your lower leg are primarily responsible for movement in your foot and ankle and also aid in bending your knee. When you point your toes, notice your calf muscle doing the work. When you flex your foot, notice the front of your shin muscles contracting.

Your Thighs are Knee Movers

The upper leg, or thigh, has two groups of very strong muscles that act on the knee. The front of your thigh has four muscles that form the quadricep group (your "quads") and is responsible primarily for straightening (extending) your leg at the knee joint. The back of your thigh has three muscles that form the hamstring group (your "hammies") and are primarily responsible for bending (flexing) your knee.

Your Hips: Your Body's Biggest Muscle

Your pelvic and buttocks muscles of your hips work to flex, extend, abduct (raise apart), adduct (bring together), and rotate your leg from the hip joint. There are three main muscles in your buttocks, known collectively as the "glutes." The Gluteus Maximus, your body's biggest muscle, is responsible for straightening (extending) your leg at the hip joint. The gluteus medius and minimus help lift (abduct) and rotate your leg to the side.

The hip flexor muscles in the front of your hip help lift your thigh and bend your leg at your hip. The inside of your leg has five muscles that originate in the hip, together called the "adductors," that help bring your legs together.

All these hip muscles help determine where your leg is in space and have an important relationship with your knee. For instance, if your gluteus medius and minimus are weak, your knees may "cave in" when you squat or sit on a chair, and that will affect the angles in your knee.

Core Muscles Are Your Trunk Stabilizers

Your core muscles are the muscles of your belly and low back. They connect your pelvis to your spine and provide stability to your entire trunk. They are like the pillar on which your shoulders and arms rest and from which your legs move.

For your lower body, if your core muscles are weak, your body may recruit your hip flexors to help stabilize your pelvis, which can cause your pelvis to rotate, which creates a chain reaction to your hamstrings.

SUMMARY

All of the muscles and joints that work together to give you movement are important to the health of your knees. The health of your knee is equally important to your other joints, from your feet to your core. Keeping all these muscles strong will help with proper body alignment and avoid compensating movements.

CHAPTER 6

THREE FACTORS FOR BEST TKR OUTCOME

TKR recovery is no joke. It is painful and emotionally draining. You'll wonder if you made the best choice. You'll wonder if you will ever sleep a full night without pain. You'll wonder if it will ever get better. And then when you start physical therapy, you'll know that your preparation, following the advice in this book and getting stronger, was well worth it. Your balance is better. You know what it feels like to use different leg muscles and understand what the PT is talking about to fire those muscles. You are focused more on reducing inflammation and increasing range of motion and not worrying as much about muscle strength because you are already strong. You have real hope that you will get through this and become even better and stronger.

The three factors for a successful TKR are: Improve Strength, Healthy Knee Movement, and Reduce the Load.

FACTOR #1: IMPROVE STRENGTH: MUSCLES, BALANCE, FLEXIBILITY

Improving strength is about strong muscles, balance, and flexibility. Being strong will help you with daily activities and the things you want to do in the world. You don't want to sit on the sidelines and let everyone else have the fun. Muscle strength, balance, and flexibility reduce your risk of falling and injury and improve your stamina and freedom of movement.

Muscle Strength

Having strong muscles will help you move more with ease. Remember how we talked about muscles as pulleys on your bones? If you have a teeny tiny pulley, it will have a much harder time pulling on the bone to create movement than if you have a bigger pulley. And don't worry about getting "bulky" with muscle—that's a hard thing to achieve even for a bodybuilder. We are focused on having good strength, starting with basic daily activities of life like lifting a box off the floor, opening heavy doors, or sitting down on and getting up from a chair without assistance. We then advance to activities like dancing, hiking, and so much more.

When you strengthen your muscles, you also strengthen your bones. Every time your muscle pulls on a bone, the bone pulls back! Thanks to Newton's 3rd Law of Motion: for every action, there is an equal and opposite reaction. That is why doctors will tell you that weight-bearing or resistance exercise (using weights or bands) is good for your bones.

Balance

Your ability to control your body in space is a matter of balance. Balance is controlled by many body systems, including your muscles, bones, joints, vision, and the balance organ in the inner ear, along with nerves, heart, and blood vessels.[23]

Getting stronger and practicing balance moves will help you in your ability to stop, start, and change directions without toppling over. Balance is an integral part of everyday movements, such as walking, running, bending over to pick up the groceries, and climbing stairs. The more you practice, the more stable you will be.

Flexibility

I like this definition of flexibility from the Oxford dictionary: "The quality of bending easily without breaking." Having muscles and joints that are flexible allows us to reach higher and bend lower without pain. Many of our muscles cross joints, so greater flexibility may offer a greater range of motion within the joint. Range of motion in your knee, however, is also determined by bones, cartilage, connective tissue, and scar tissue. For example, if you have tight hamstrings, you may not be able to straighten your leg fully when hinged at the hips. If you have tight quadricep muscles, they may limit how far you can bend your knees. If you are tight through any of your hip muscles, you may have a limited range of motion while lifting your leg and bending at your hips. If you cannot lift the ball of your foot off the ground very far or have restrictions in your ankle, it will affect how deep you can go in your squat.

---

23 Mayo Clinic, 2018. "Balance Problems." Accessed February 12, 2020. https://www.mayoclinic.org/diseases-conditions/balance-problems/symptoms-causes/syc-20350474

Regularly stretching your muscles will help you feel more nimble and able. Dynamic stretching involves movement while performing the stretch and is an excellent warm-up before your workout or just to start your day. Static stretching involves holding a pose for an extended period (30 seconds or more) and is best done after your muscles are warm, such as during your cool down from your workout.

FACTOR #2: HEALTHY KNEE MOVEMENT: "OIL YOUR JOINT"

When your knee hurts, moving it is not necessarily the first thing you think of. Any achy or painful knee can start to feel and act like a rusty hinge. The less you move it, the harder it becomes to move. What you need is some "oil" for your joint.

The good news is that you already have the "oil," it just may be in poor shape. Your knee joint capsule has synovial fluid, which reduces the friction between bones and nourishes cartilage. Healthy synovial fluid is viscous (thick), sort of like raw egg white. Inflammation and oxidation stress cause synovial fluid to become thinner and less able to lubricate, which can lead to several joint diseases.[24]

When your knee joint is at rest, your cartilage absorbs some of the synovial fluid. When the joint is in use, some of that synovial fluid is squeezed out of the cartilage—like wringing water from

---

24 *Interdisciplinary Toxicology*, 2013. "Hyaluronan and synovial joint: function, distribution, and healing." Accessed February 14, 2020. https://www.ncbi.nlm.nih.gov/pmc/articles/PMC3967437/

a sponge—and circulates through the joint.[25] Moving your knee through the right kind of exercise will help your synovial fluid do a better job of lubricating, nourishing cartilage, and reducing your knee pain.

You can see why it makes sense to move your knee more. Now, the question is how to do this without causing pain? There are three keys to this answer: No weight-bearing, no impact, and no lateral movement.

No Weight Bearing

For your knees, weight bearing exercise means that your feet are carrying the weight of your body. Carrying the weight of your body through your feet and knees can add up to more pain, and running, walking, or even standing can be uncomfortable. The more you weigh, the higher the burden on your knees.

There are several exercise options that are good for your knees and remove the weight from your feet:
- Cycling (upright or recumbent bikes)
- Swimming
- Rowing Machine (or rowing outdoor in a skull)
- Strength Training Options

Of these options, cycling is the one I recommend the most because your knee is repeating the full range of motion. Knee range of motion to pedal a bike is about 110 degrees. All of your body weight

25 Arthritis-health.com, 2 016. "How do Synovial Joints Work?" Accessed February 14, 2020. https://www.arthritis-health.com/types/joint-anatomy/how-do-synovial-joints-work.

is supported by the seat of the bike. Plus, people commonly have access to a bike to ride outside or a stationary bike.

Swimming is a wonderful option because the water is supporting your entire body weight and providing resistance to your movement. Your knee uses a lower range of motion than cycling, but you are still using the kicking action, which is good for your knee. By the way, some programs combine bicycling and water, commonly called "aqua-cycling," where the bike is in the water.

The rowing machine seat supports your body weight, and the rowing action uses not only your legs but involves your arms and core for a full-body workout. Knee range of motion required for a rowing machine is in the average range of 105-120 degrees.[26]

Strength training with no weight bearing would mean that you are sitting or lying down as you do the exercise. There are many options for this, but none as repetitive as cycling, swimming, and rowing. I definitely recommend strength training as a supplement to these.

No Impact

What does this mean, exactly? Consider that each time you take a step while walking (or running), your heels—along with your ankles, knees, and hip joints—absorb the force of your body weight, plus the effects of gravity. Remember the discussion earlier about impact forces? Each time your foot hits the ground when you're running, it can impart a force up to 4-14 times your body weight.

---

26 Journal of Human Kinetics, 2013. "A Physiological and Kinematic Comparison of Two Different Lean Back Positions During Stationary Rowing On a Concept II Machine." Accessed March 24, 2020. https://www.ncbi.nlm.nih.gov/pmc/articles/PMC3796848/

Your joints absorb this force. The knee catches the largest portion since it has the greatest movement.

Activities are considered to be "no-impact" when there is no repeated foot strike with the ground. There will be some compression in the joints caused by the movements, but the percussive heel strike has been removed. This is good, especially for painful or arthritic joints, and good for maintaining the health of your replacement joint. Impact activities are not recommended for total knee replacements.

Every time you have an impact-caused compression, the bones in your knees come closer together. If your knee joint is healthy, this impact is no problem because your cartilage is doing its job as your knee's shock absorber. However, if you are missing cartilage, have arthritic changes in your knee, or have an issue with your ligaments or tendons, impact activities may cause more wear-and-tear in the joint. The same is true once you replace your knee. Over time, the jarring from impact can loosen the implants and cause pain or even lead to the necessity of a revision. The plastic meniscus replacement, as a part of your new joint, can also become worn out.

No and low impact activities that are great for your knees include:
- Cycling (upright or recumbent bikes)
- Swimming
- Rowing Machine (or outdoor rowing in a skull)
- Elliptical Machine (foot stays in contact with the tread for full stride)
- Stair Machine (only if going upstairs does not currently hurt your knees)

No Lateral Movement

Lateral movement refers to side-to-side movements of your knees, such as shuffle steps in basketball or carving turns in downhill skiing. Lateral movement is the source of much knee damage and pain. If you have pain with lateral movement, try these exercises that are good for your knees:

- Cycling (stationary or outdoor bike)
- Elliptical Machine
- Rowing Machine
- Stair Machine
- Swimming*

I put an *asterisk by "swimming" because if you are kicking in the water and you have some laxity in your knee ligaments, you may feel an uncomfortable wobble in your knee as you kick. This was my case, and my knee would hurt more after swimming. There is very minor lateral knee movement in the other exercises listed. The straightforward knee path keeps your knees in proper alignment without any of the potentially irritating side-to-side movement.

Choose the exercise that suits you the best: it's a win-win-win if you choose one that offers all three benefits of no impact, no weight-bearing, and no lateral movement. From our exercises above, that narrows the list to cycling and using a rowing machine.

Through my 12 knee surgeries, riding a bike has always been my go-to activity. In fact, until I finally had both knees replaced, I felt more comfortable on a bike than I did on my own two feet. I like to joke that instead of being a biped, I'm a two-wheeler. Bicycling has brought great joy to my life, from the exhilaration of riding my one-speed bike with a basket around my neighborhood to the complete freedom, independence, and sense of accomplishment that comes with bicycle adventures and pedaling to new and unknown places all under my own power. Plus, indoor cycling allows me to ramp my intensity to go easy or hard, focus on specific training parameters, generate endorphins (natural feel-good and happiness brain chemicals). In the last few years, I have kept an online journal about my bicycle travels, and I invite you to read them at www.healthykneescoach.com/blog. Go back to 6/18/17 for the beginning of the adventure. I hope my journal will inspire you to try bicycling in whatever form you can.

FACTOR #3: REDUCE THE LOAD AND YOU'LL DECREASE STRESS

We talked about weight-bearing and that your body weight is magnified as force through your knee on every step. You can do something that will help decrease this stress: shave off any excess weight you have. If you are overweight, your doctor may have mentioned this to you already for the sake of your knees. If you are obese, your doctor may even require you to lose weight before they perform a total knee replacement. Even if you are carrying just ten extra pounds, that will make 20-30 pounds more force in your knee on every step. I repeat this because it is so important for your knee health to drop off extra pounds.

To lose one pound of fat, you must create a deficit of 3500 calories. This can be done either through calorie restriction (eat fewer calories) or increased exercise (burn more calories). To lose weight, a combination of some of each is recommended: Gain muscle to boost your metabolism, exercise to burn calories, and reduce caloric intake while eating high-quality food.

Increase Your Body's Demand for Calories

As you gain lean muscle mass, you will give a boost to your metabolism and increase your body's demand for calories. Adding more muscle means your body has a higher need for fuel, and your basic requirement for calories will go up. That means you burn more calories at rest in order to fuel more muscle, and this may help you lose some fat.

Burn More Calories

Adding exercise to your daily routine will help you create the caloric deficit you need to lose weight. Here are some of the most common forms of exercise that are easier on your knees and their average calorie expenditures. Every person is different, so these numbers are just estimates:

Typical Calorie Expenditures for Exercise:[27]

Activity (1-hour duration)	Calorie Expenditure (160 lb person)
Aerobics, low-impact	365
Aerobics, water	402
Bicycling < 10mph, leisure	290
Bicycling 12-13.9 mph, moderate	580
Dancing, ballroom	219

---

27 Mayo Clinic, 2019. "Exercise for Weight Loss: Calories Burned in 1 Hour." Accessed March 6, 2020. https://www.mayoclinic.org/healthy-lifestyle/weight-loss/in-depth/exercise/art-20050999. Supplemented with additional information from the original 2011 study, "Compendium of Physical Activities." Accessed March 6, 2020. https://sites.google.com/site/compendiumofphysicalactivities/home.

Activity (1-hour duration)	Calorie Expenditure (160 lb person)
Elliptical trainer, moderate	365
Rowing (100 Watts)	537
Rowing (150 Watts)	652
Stair Machine	690
Swimming laps, moderate	423
Walking, 3.5mph	314

Reduce Calorie Intake and Eat Higher Quality Food

A simple way to get started losing weight is to rearrange your plate. A more in-depth discussion of this follows in the "Eat Smarter: Prepare for and Recover from Surgery Faster with the Right Nutrition" section, but it's also one of the key factors in your best TKR outcome.

You probably already know a few things you could do to clean up your eating habits. Take one day at a time and do your best. There are some good rules of thumb to follow that lead to smart choices for your foods:

- Make half your plate fruits or vegetables
- Reduce or eliminate processed (packaged) foods
- Eat more fresh foods
- Cut down on sweets
- Cut back or eliminate alcohol consumption or at least switch to "lite"
- Choose a clear broth instead of a creamy one
- Choose grilled meats over fried

- Skip the heavy cream sauces
- Eat slowly and eat until you are satisfied, not bursting
- Throughout the day, drink half your body weight in water ounces (if you weigh 200 pounds, drink 100 oz of water). Drink an additional 20 oz of water for every hour you exercise.

To sum it up, the three factors that will help set you up for a quicker recovery from your surgery are Improve Strength, Healthy Knee Movement, and Reduce the Load. Now you know the why, so let's get to the how with our 5 Pillar Plan that will get you ready for surgery and help your outcome be all the things you hope for.

CHAPTER 7

HOW TO TRAIN LIKE AN ATHLETE WITH THE 5 PILLAR PLAN

OK, Team, here we go! I've shared with you the "why" of what you'll want to do to prepare for and continue recovery from your TKR. Now let's get to the specifics of what to do. The stretches, exercises, dietary recommendations, and mental "hacks" in this chapter are the pillars for you to influence the outcome of your surgery, feel stronger, and return to an active life.

Approach this like an athlete with an exercise plan. Eat well to support the demands of your body with the stresses of surgery and maintain a positive goal-oriented attitude.

Here are the five pillars of the plan that will help you prepare for and recover faster from your total knee replacement:

1. **Get Stronger:** Improve Muscle Strength and Balance
2. **Move More:** Ride a Bike the Right Way
3. **Get Flexible:** Practice Stretch and Release Techniques
4. **Eat Smarter:** Prepare for and Recover from Surgery Faster with the Right Nutrition
5. **Right Mind:** Consistency and Positive Attitude

PILLAR #1 GET STRONGER: IMPROVE MUSCLE STRENGTH AND BALANCE

The exercises presented here can be used two ways: to prepare before surgery and to continue with strengthening after your post-surgery physical therapy is complete. They are both important, and the latter is often ignored. Continuing on with exercises to support the strength of your legs will bring you the best on-going results. This is a life-long endeavor.

There are hundreds of exercises you *could* do and get lost in all the options. I've made this simple for you with a select list of the most important exercises to do in preparation for and continuing a strong recovery from your TKR.

Don't worry; strength is not about showy muscles. Strength is about independence. It's about getting on and off the floor without needing help. It's about keeping your balance when you trip. It's about climbing the Spanish Steps with confidence on the trip of a lifetime in Rome (or wherever your heart takes you). It's about being confident that your body is strong and ready for action.

Gaining strength will give you more control, help with reducing compensations due to muscle imbalances, and help boost your metabolism by building more muscle. Resistance training will not only help your muscles get stronger but will help your bones get stronger too.

To get stronger, there are three key elements to keep your knees in top working condition: Movement Foundations, Balance Training, and Strength Training. For a free guide with pictures of every move, please go to www.healthykneescoach.com/HKstrength.

Use these basic rules:
- Repeat each exercise 5-10X. When you can repeat 10X easily, try the "Advance this Move" option if there is one.
- To advance a move that uses dumbbells, increase weight by no more than 10%.
- Slower is better. Make each move slowly and with control.

MOVEMENT FOUNDATIONS
Movement Foundations start with the essential elements that are the foundations for healthy movement. We will work to break apart compensating actions, stop bad habits, and stimulate control.

There are Seven Movement Foundations:
- Short Foot
- Pelvic Tilts
- Abdominal Bracing
- Belly Breathing
- Glute Pops and Quad Squeezes
- Knee Knockouts
- Elements of the Squat

Movement Foundation #1: Short Foot

Purpose: Short Foot exercises are used to strengthen the foot muscles (especially the arch) and improve your balance.[28] If the arch of your foot collapses, it follows that your knees may become knock-kneed (or valgus).

How to: Best done barefoot, while seated or standing, grip the floor with your toes and lift up with your arch—like you are trying to lift your arch while pressing your heel and toes into the floor. If you look at your bare foot while doing this, your foot actually appears a little shorter (thus the name).

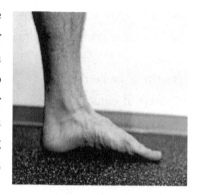

It is not a big movement but will work to strengthen foot muscles and improve leg alignment and balance.

Movement Foundation #2: Pelvic Tilts

Purpose: Pelvic tilts serve as a good educational exercise, teaching you to feel your abdominals and their actions better. This will allow you to better utilize them during exercise. This exercise also helps to correct for anterior pelvic tilt, where the hip flexors are

---

28 US National Library of Medicine, National Institutes of Health, 2019. "Short-Foot Exercise Promotes Quantitative Somatosensory Function in Ankle Instability: a Randomized Controlled Trial." Accessed December 18, 2019. https://www.ncbi.nlm.nih.gov/pmc/articles/PMC6350454/

shortened, and hip extensors are lengthened, causing an excessive curvature of the low back.

How to (Standing): Stand with your feet hip-distance apart and relax your spine. Place your hands on your hips and rock your pelvis forward (to create more of an arch in your low back), then rock your pelvis back (to create less of an arch in your low back).

How to (Lying on the Floor): Lying face-up, with your knees bent and your feet flat on the floor, place your hands under your low back. Using your hips and abdominals, press your low back into your hands or the floor. You'll feel like you are rocking your pelvis. Now release the pressure and create a small arch in your back by pressing your pelvis down toward your buttocks.

Movement Foundation #3: Abdominal Bracing

Purpose: We want to help you understand where your core muscles are located, so you have better control of them. Abdominal bracing is all about contracting your core muscles like you are bracing yourself against someone who is going to tickle you! As you do this, you create a natural belt or girdle that protects you. The muscles involved are the transversus abdominis, the rectus abdominus, the internal and external obliques, the pelvic floor muscles, and the multifidus muscle.

How to: While standing with feet hip-width apart, squeeze or suck in your belly as if someone is going to tickle you. At the same time, suck up the floor of your pelvis as if you are guarding, or pulling up, your private parts (the same feeling as doing a "Kegel").

Movement Foundation #4: Belly Breathing

Purpose: Do you ever think about your breathing? How we breathe makes a difference, especially during exercise. We want you to become aware of your breath and how you can shift from shallow breaths in your chest to deep ones in your belly.

When you breathe through your nose, your olfactory nerves (which dangle in your sinus cavities) are stimulated to signal to your brain that oxygen is coming in, and you will naturally take a deeper breath. This is not true for mouth breathing. So, training yourself to breathe deep will help in many parts of your life, from exercise to stress relief.

How to: Place your hands on your chest and take a breath in through your mouth, visualizing that you are breathing into your hands. Now, place your hands on your belly and take a deep breath through your nose and notice how your belly expands and the breath feels deeper than when you had your hands on your chest. Exhale through your mouth.

Next, keep your hands on your belly and try to replicate that deep breath while breathing through your mouth. Use this technique to train your breathing to be nice and deep, no matter if you take in your breath through your nose or your mouth.

Movement Foundation #5: Glute Pops and Quad Squeezes

No, these are not summer-time desserts; they are exercises that you can do anytime. They will likely be a part of your TKR post-surgery recovery. So, it is best to start them beforehand so that you know just what they feel like and can get your muscles responding a little faster afterward.

Purpose: Let's make sure that you understand how to engage certain muscles: your gluteus maximus (buttocks or butt) and quadricep (front of thigh) groups. With knee injuries or post-knee surgery, sometimes it's a little bit harder to "connect" with these muscles. We want to make sure that you are in control.

How to Glute Pops (Seated or Lying Down): Starting in a chair or on the floor with legs straight, squeeze your butt (gluteus maximus), and you should feel your hips rise. Try squeezing only one side and then the other.

How to Quad Squeeze: Sitting on the floor, place a rolled-up towel or foam roller under one knee. Now squeeze your thigh (quadricep), so your leg straightens. Repeat on the other leg.

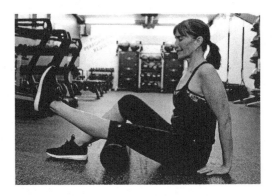

Movement Foundation #6: Knee Knockouts

Purpose: Knee knockouts work on hip stability and gluteus minimus and medius strength (side butt muscles).

How to: With a mini band around your knees, assume a stance slightly wider than hip-width. Pivot your knee in and then out with a slight movement in the foot like you are squishing a bug, with the movement being produced from your hip.

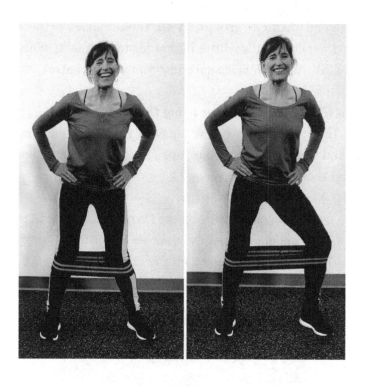

Movement Foundation #7: Elements of the Squat

So many folks with knee issues are scared of squats, and I can understand why—because they can hurt! But they don't have to, and we hope to show you how best to squat for your body. Even before your TKR, try these moves to see if you can begin to retrain your body for proper squat mechanics. Only go as low as your knee pain will allow. Post TKR (once you are recovered), there should be no knee pain associated with a squat.

Purpose: Every time you sit on a chair, you are performing a squat. Squats are a needed movement for everyday living. Learning to perform them properly, so you do not experience knee pain can be life-changing!

How to: We like to break down the squat into a flow of three pieces: hip hinge, knee bend, and open chest with flat back. Start with your hands pressed together in front of you and your feet around hip-width apart. It is important to note that feet hip-width apart is just a societal "normal." It is a good starting position, but many people will require a wider or narrower squat stance to pro-

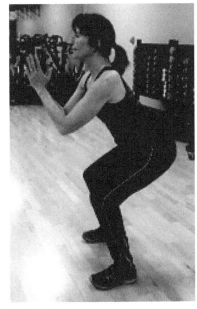

mote proper depth, comfort, and performance. Play around with the width of your feet, and how pointed out your toes are to find the most comfortable position for you and your knees.

Feet can be pointing forward or slightly to the sides—whatever is more comfortable for you. Start with bending (hinging) at the hips first, then bending the knees to lower to the floor, while keeping the chest open with a flat back and eyes on the horizon. Really push your booty out behind you! This avoids premature forward movement of the knee by shifting the hips backward.

BALANCE TRAINING

No one wants to fall, right? Working on your body's ability to balance will help prevent fall-related injuries, correct for some compensations, and improve your kinesthetic awareness of your body in three-dimensional space.

Balance training includes not only the ability to stand on one leg but also to control your body as you change direction and start and stop movement. Your body has mass, and when the mass is in motion, it takes the coordination of your muscles to affect which direction your body is moving. Balance is a huge part of this. Balance training should be done on each leg, even if one is weaker than the other.

There are two essential balance training moves for you, with challenges and advancements for each:

- Tandem Balance
- Single Leg

Balance Training #1: Tandem Balance

Purpose: The Tandem Balance takes your normal wide stance (feet under hips) and makes it narrow (feet in alignment with heel touching toe) in order to work on balance. Work up to holding this balance for 30-60 seconds. Do the same with the opposite foot in front.

How to Tandem Balance (With Support) Start: Stand near a wall and use one hand to gently support yourself as you get the feeling for this balance move. Place equal weight on each foot with your feet lined up heel to toe.

How to Tandem Balance (Without Support) Advance 1: While standing, place one foot directly in alignment with the other with heel touching toe. Place equal weight on each foot. Then shift weight forward to put more weight on the forward leg and shift weight backward to place more weight on the back leg. Rock back and forth, pausing with balance on each leg.

How to Tandem Balance (With Head-Turning) Advance 2: Once you feel balanced without support, with your eyes open, try turning your head to look over your right shoulder, then over your left.

How to Tandem Balance (With Eyes Closed) Advance 3: Go back to the (actual) corner for this. Align your feet, get balanced, then close your eyes, and maintain your balance.

How to Tandem Balance (Walking Movement) Advance 4: With your right foot planted, move your left foot in front, get balanced, then move your left foot behind, get balanced. Change to your left foot planted with rotating your right foot in front and in back. Then keep advancing with several steps forward followed by several steps backward. When all of that feels steady, rotate your head to look left and right as you step.

Balance Training #2: Single Leg

Purpose: To further challenge your balance, we narrow your base of support to one leg, not two. Balance training is an easy thing to incorporate in daily activities. For instance, while waiting in line for groceries (or any line, really), simply shift your weight from one leg to the other, moving to single-leg stance, holding it on each leg.

How to Single Leg (With Support) Start: With your hand supported on a wall, a table, or a chair, shift your weight to the supporting leg and lift the other foot off the ground. Try to reduce the amount of support you need so you can balance while standing on just one leg.

How to Single Leg (No Support) Advance 1: Press your hands together in front of you, shift your weight to your supporting leg, and lift one foot off the ground.

For one-minute, alternate standing single leg for 10 seconds per leg, then advance to 15 seconds per leg, 20 seconds, and so on until you can stand for one minute per leg without support.

How to Single Leg (While Brushing Teeth) Advance 2: The best way to form a new habit is to tack it onto an existing one like brushing your teeth. Stand on one leg while you brush your lowers, then switch the other leg while you brush your uppers. This is an easy way to incorporate balance twice a day. The wiggling and jiggling while you brush helps to fine-tune your balancing muscles.

How to Single Leg (Leg Swings) Advance 3: By moving your free leg, you change your center of gravity, and that recruits more neuromuscular control to maintain balance.

While standing on one leg, slowly swing your free leg forward, out to the side, and backward. Create your own swing patterns to challenge your balance.

How to Single Leg (Tree Pose) Advance 4: By changing your center of gravity with your leg position, you challenge your ability to balance.

With your hands pressed together in front of you, shift your weight to one leg. Then lift the other foot and place it as high as you can on the inner leg calf or above your knee on the thigh of your supporting leg. Check your posture; stand up tall!

STRENGTH TRAINING

Making your muscles stronger is the key to freedom of movement. Remember, your bones are your framework, and your muscles are the pulleys that move the bones to create movement. If your muscles are weak, your movement will be more difficult and can be harder on your joints. Strong muscles equal easier and more balanced movement.

There are four predominant areas to strengthen in order to have healthy knees:

- Knee Dominant
- Hip Dominant
- Ankle and Calf
- Core

Equipment:

To make it a little easier for you, we have put together a kit with the equipment shown below. You can purchase this kit from HealthyKneesCoach.com/shop.

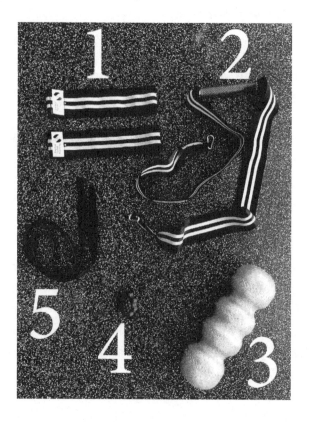

1. **Mini-Band**—A small circular band that can stretch to about two times its length. It comes in a variety of materials. Our favorite is the wider elastic band shown in the picture (from Anchor Point Training) because it will not curl up as you put it on. The bands often come in various sizes or different levels of resistance.

2. **Suspension Strap**—A thick elastic band with hooks on each end and a handle that slides to adjust along the strap. The band attaches to a door strap (#5 in the picture), which keeps it secure. The "anchor point" refers to where the suspension strap is attached to the door. Directions for using the suspension strap usually call for "facing the anchor point" (meaning the front of your body is facing the point where the Suspension Strap is fastened to the door) or "facing away from the anchor point" (meaning the anchor point is behind you).

3. **Foam Roller**—Usually a long cylinder of 4-inch diameter, made of a dense molded poly material. It comes in a variety of lengths from about 18 inches to 48 inches. The Rollga foam roller shown here is shaped for more support to your muscles as you roll.

4. **Helo Massage Ball**—The Rollga Helo Massage Ball uses neuro activators (rough bumps designed to grab skin) on one side, and a round lacrosse ball feature on the opposite side to both stimulate fascia and unlock tension and stress. Additionally, tiny nodes or 'fingers' fill the circumference of the ball and are designed to pinpoint trigger points and address fascial scaring. The Helo Massage Ball takes the premise of a lacrosse ball and adds three more recovery friendly applications. We use this ball for the Piriformis Release.

5. **Door Strap**—This strap allows you to connect the Suspension Strap to any standard door.

Not Pictured:

6. **Dumbbell**—A short bar with a weight at each end and comes in a variety of weights. If you don't have dumbbells at home, you can hold anything heavy, like a bag filled with books, to create the extra resistance. You can also use a weighted ball for many of the exercises

7. **Chair, Plyobox, Weight Bench**—We do sit-to-stand exercises, so you'll need something to sit on! If a chair or weight bench seems too low, try using a higher Plyobox at your fitness club, or a sturdy tabletop or your bed at home.

8. **Rolled Up Towel**—(for stretching assists and quadricep engagement exercises)

9. **Foam Pad**—A thick square of foam to give some cushion to your knees when kneeling or can be used for standing balance challenges.

Strength Training #1: Knee Dominant (KD)

Knee Dominant exercises directly work the muscles affecting the knee, primarily your quadriceps and hamstring groups.

KD 1: Terminal Knee Extension

Purpose: This exercise focuses on control of your quadricep muscles with concentric (contraction) and eccentric (release of the contraction) movements.

How to: Attach a mini-band around the suspension strap attached high and low on a door or slip the mini-band around a stable table leg. Place one leg inside the loop with the band at your knee and face the anchor point. Stand far enough away to create tension on the band at the back of your knee. Allow the banded knee to bend with control as the band pulls it forward. Then squeeze your quadricep muscles as you straighten your leg at the knee.

KD 2: Squat Preparation

Purpose: I didn't want to scare you with the word "squat," so I added in "preparation"—but remember, you squat every day when you sit down and rise from a chair (or the toilet). These exercises are designed to strengthen your legs so you can be confident and then even powerful in your ability to squat anytime.

How to Squat Preparation (Wall Slides) Start: While leaning with your back against a wall and feet about 2-foot lengths in front of the wall, slide down the wall until you come close to a "sitting" position. The goal is to get your thighs parallel to the floor, but it may take some practice before you can do this. Adjust your feet so your knees do not slide in front of your toes. Slide down only as far as is comfortable. Hold the sitting position for 5 seconds then slide up the wall to return to standing. (If your knees hurt during this move, try moving your feet closer or further away from the wall or taking a wider or narrower stance.)

This is an exercise favored by skiers to strengthen quad endurance. You can start with just a 5 second hold and work up to a minute.

How to Squat Preparation (Anchor Point Supported Squat) Advance: Hook both ends of the Anchor Suspension Strap at the top of the door. Grip the handle with elbows at your side while facing the door and creating tension on the strap.

Lower into a squat position by using the elements of a squat discussed earlier: bend at the hips, keep a flat back and your chest pointing at the wall (not at the floor). Then bend your knees as your hips push behind you. Only go as low as tolerated by any knee pain. As you rise back to standing, press through your heels, and use your arms to assist you as much as you need.

How to Squat Preparation (Sit to Stand) Advance 2: The sit-to-stand move is what you do every day. I want to help you to feel strong and confident prior to TKR. You will need to rely on your non-operated leg a lot after surgery, and we want you strong and ready for that.

Sit to Stand #1 (With Counterbalance Weight): Use a weight, such as a dumbbell, weighted ball, or some heavy object that you can hold. Start standing with your feet shoulder-width apart and a bit in front of the chair (or bench or plyobox) you are going to sit on.

Hold the dumbbell weight at chest height, then press the weight forward as you hinge your hips back and lower toward the chair.

From the seated position, start with the weight held at arm's length at chest height, then bring the weight back toward your chest as you rise to stand. As you get stronger, you'll use a lower and lower weight to assist.

Sit to Stand #2: (No Counterbalance): Do the sit to stand without a dumbbell weight. Do not use your hands to push off from the chair.

Sit to Stand #3 (Body Weight): Remove the chair! Just lower into a squat position, then return to standing.

Sit to Stand #4 (Goblet Squat): With a goblet squat, not only are you working on your legs and tush, but also your arms, shoulders, and core as you hold and stabilize the weight.

Hold a dumbbell vertically with your hands cupping the top end of the weight like you are holding a big goblet with the heels of your hands. Hold this weight at high chest level, with elbows pinned at your rib cage. Feet are about hip-width apart, toes pointed forward or slightly out.

Keeping your arms close to your chest and elbows pointing down, bend your hips, then knees, to lower your body into a squat position, as low as you can comfortably go over about 3-5 seconds. When you return to standing, drive through your glutes, legs, and heels to return to starting position, over about 3-5 seconds. Maintain control in both down and upward movements.

Strength Training #2: Hip Dominant (HD)

The Hip Dominant exercises directly affect the hip joint. Since the thigh bone (femur) is also part of your knee joint, what happens at the hip affects the knee.

There are three primary moves:
- Hip Extension
- Side Leg Lifts
- Hip Hinge (to deadlifts)

HD 1: Hip Extension

Purpose: The hip extension helps to strengthen your posterior chain (the back of your leg) with emphasis on your big butt muscle, the gluteus maximus, with help from the hamstrings.

The hip extension is most effectively done from the floor, but I've included a standing option if getting down to the floor and back up again is a little too much for you right now. If you can get on and off the floor, please start with the Glute Bridge.

How to Hip Extension (Standing Option): Stand erect, facing a wall or chair. Support yourself with both hands on the wall or the back of a chair. Squeeze your butt and raise one leg slightly backward, keeping your knee straight. Be mindful to keep your hips stable and do not arch your back. Your foot may only arc about three to four inches off the floor.

How to Hip Extension (Glute Bridge): Lie face up on the floor, knees bent and feet flat on the floor, heels as close to your booty as you can. Place your hands on the floor, palms down next to your hips. Exhale, squeeze your butt, and lift your hips off the ground so that you form a straight line from knees to shoulders. Inhale as you return your hips to the ground. Do both motions slowly and with control. As you get stronger, hold the hip lifted position for a five-count.

If you notice that your knees dip together during the hip bridge, place a mini-band around your legs, just above your knees. Perform the exercise while keeping tension on the mini-band, not allowing it to go slack as you raise your hips.

HD 2: Side Leg

Purpose: Remember, the gluteus medius and minimus are muscles beneath and to the side of the gluteus maximus. These are important muscles that help stabilize the pelvis and are the prime movers and controllers for side leg movement.

You'll start exercising them with bodyweight only. When this is easy, add resistance by placing a mini band around both legs just above your knees. The closer you slide the mini band toward your ankles, the more challenging this move will become. When the mini band is placed below your knees, it will create lateral force at the knee joint, primarily on the lifting leg. If this causes you pain, keep the mini band at or above your knee. This lateral force in the knee joint is a good way to help strengthen your collateral ligaments.

How to Side Leg (Weight Shifts) Start: Standing with feet shoulder-width apart, your goal is to keep your legs the same distance apart as you rock to one leg and lift the other off the floor. Add a mini-band around both legs to add a challenge.

How to Side Leg Lifts (Standing): Stand side facing to a wall with the closest hand for support, the other hand on your hip. With your knee straight and your toes pointed forward (not up!), exhale as you raise your leg to the side. Do not shift your hips as you do this exercise. Inhale as you return your leg to the start position.

How to Side Leg Lifts (Side Lying on Floor): Lie down on your side with legs extended and stacked so that your body is in a straight line. Slightly bend your bottom leg for support. With toes pointed forward, exhale as you lift your top leg slightly behind you. Inhale as you return your leg to the stacked position.

Are you doing it right? If you feel the work happening in your quadriceps, your toes are pointing up. You need to point your toes forward or even a little down. You should definitely feel the work in your side butt.

HD 3: Hip Hinge (to deadlifts)

Purpose: The hip hinge movement is key for squats and deadlifts. We've already covered squats a few times, and now we will work our way toward a deadlift. You will be amazed at how powerful you feel!

The hip hinge primarily targets your "backside" or posterior chain, with your glutes, hamstrings, and low back.

How to Hip Hinge (Supported) Start: With both ends of the anchor point suspension strap hooked at the top of the door, stand facing the anchor point with your arms straight and hands pressing down on the handle. Keep your feet about shoulder-width apart and a slight bend in your knees. Inhale as you bend forward with a flat back, pushing your hips back and surfing your hands forward. To return to standing, exhale as you push your hips forward, keeping the downward tension on the handle. As you return to standing, focus on your hips pressing forward, not your back lifting up.

How to Hip Hinge (Good Mornings) Advance 1: Start standing with your feet shoulder-width apart and place your hands on your chest. Use good posture with shoulders back and brace your abdominals. Inhale as you hinge forward at your hips, pushing your booty behind. Have a slight bend in your knees. Try to create a 90-degree hinge, so your torso is parallel to the floor. Exhale as you return to standing.

To make this move a little more challenging, change your center of gravity by placing your hands behind your head.

How to Hip Hinge (Deadlifts) Advance 2: The deadlift directly targets all of the major muscle groups responsible for correct posture, core strength, and leg power. The primary muscle groups include gluteus maximus (butt), hamstrings (back of thigh), quadriceps (front of thigh), extensor spinae (low back), trapezius (upper back) and many other supporting muscles from your calves to core.

The key to success with the deadlift is to start with a light weight so you have the proper form before going to a heavier weight.

Stand erect with your feet slightly wider than shoulder-width apart, with a slight bend in your knees. Hold your weight (dumbbell, barbell, kettlebell) close to your body. Exhale as you hinge at your hips, with a flat back and neutral neck, lower the weight toward your knees, allowing your knees to bend slightly while keeping hips high. Exhale as you return to standing while keeping the weight close to your legs.

Strength Training #3: Ankle and Calf (AC)

Your lower legs are primarily responsible for how your feet move, but also have a role in "unlocking" the knees from their straight position. Remember, your knee health is a symphony of movement starting from your feet.

Your calves (gastrocnemius and soleus) help bend your knees and lift the heel, creating plantar flexion. The fronts of your shins (tibialis anterior) help control the lift up of the top of your foot (dorsiflexion). Strengthening your lower leg muscles will help give you more control of leg movement, and that is good for your knees!

We'll focus on three main exercises:
- Ankle Mobility
- Dorsiflexion
- Plantar Flexion

AC 1: Ankle Mobility
Purpose: Ankle mobility exercises work on ankle range of motion and strength of your ankle extensor and flexor muscles.

This is a great exercise to get in the habit of doing while you are sitting down relaxing, maybe even watching TV.

How to: Lift one foot off the floor and draw the alphabet with your toes. This is working on ankle mobility and strength. Repeat on the other foot. For an added challenge, draw the alphabet in reverse (Z to A)—great for your ankle, great for your brain.

AC 2: Dorsiflexion: Toe Tappers

Purpose: This exercise focuses primarily on the range of motion and muscles that lift the top of your foot and will aid in your ability to squat.

When you lift the top of your foot closer toward your shin, that is called dorsi (top of foot) flexion (bending at the ankle).

How to: Sitting, with your feet on the floor, keep your heel on the floor while you lift the ball of your foot as high as you can, then return to the floor like you are tapping your foot. Be intentional here by lifting the ball of your foot as high as you can between taps. You can tap one foot at a time, or both, or alternate.

AC 3: Plantar Flexion: Heel Raise

Purpose: Heel raises will help strengthen your calf muscles which help your foundation—your ankles and feet—to become more stable. "Plantar" refers to the bottom of your foot. Plantar flexion, then, means bringing the bottom of the foot closer to the back of your leg by straightening your ankle (pointing your toes).

How to Heel Raise Start: At first, stand near a wall for balance. With your feet hip-width apart, lift your heels off the floor while pressing into the balls of both feet. Keep good posture with abdominal muscles pulled in so that as you lift your heels, your body shifts upward rather than forward or backward. Check your heels: if they roll out when you raise up, place a tennis ball between your ankles and hold it there while you raise and lower. This is one of our favorite moves to practice while standing in line at the grocery store (minus the tennis ball).

How to Heel Raise (Unsupported) Advance 1: Next try the heel raises without support from the wall.

How to Heel Raise (With Weights) Advance 2: Hold dumbbells at your side to increase the resistance and balance challenge.

How to Heel Raise and Drop (On Stair) Advance 3: Standing with the balls of your feet on a stair, allow your heels to drop lower than the stair, then press up to the balls of your feet. Hold onto the stair rail or balance on the wall, do this one slowly and with control as you stretch your calf muscles with the heel drop.

How to Heel Raise (Single Leg Supported) Advance 4: Using a wall for stability, balance on one leg and raise your heel. When you feel confident, try this move without support.

Strength Training #4: Core (CO)

Strengthening your core muscles is important for the stabilization of your hips and spine.

There are thousands of core strengthening moves, so we have selected a few that can be done standing. Others will require getting on hands and knees on the floor. If knees on the floor is a challenge for you, try kneeling on a foam pad to give a little more cushion and support.

There are several advancements for each move. Do not move on to the more difficult one until you have mastered the first move.

CO 1: Anti-Rotation: Pallof Press

Purpose: The Pallof Press (named after physical therapist John Pallof) is an anti-rotation exercise that strengthens core muscles that help protect your low back.

How to: Connect your anchor point strap at the top and bottom of the door and adjust the handle, so it is chest high when you have tension on the strap. Start side facing to the door in an athletic position (feet shoulder-width apart, slight bend in knees, chest up) with tension on the band. Grab the band handle with both hands and bring it to your chest. There should be tension on the band.

Exhale and press the handle straight forward. Resist the pull of the band toward the attachment—this is the "anti-rotation" part of the exercise. Return the handles to your chest.

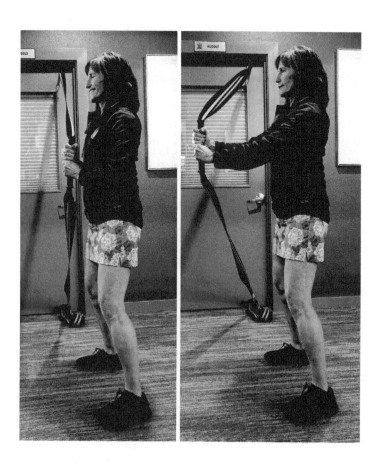

Pallof Press Variations:

- Pallof Press with 5-second hold
- Pallof Press with stir the pot: hold the handle at chest height and make a big circle as you press the handle away and return to your chest like you are stirring a big cauldron.
- Narrow your foot stance (bring feet closer together)
- Change feet to a lunge stance (one foot forward, one back)
- Pallof Press—walk out: as you are holding the press, take a step away from the anchor point, hold, and step back in.

CO 2: Suitcase Hold

Purpose: The Suitcase Hold is a basic, but very functional exercise that not only strengthens the core, but also targets shoulders, upper back, arms, legs, and grip strength.

How to: Use a dumbbell or kettlebell (or a heavy suitcase!) with one hand. Choose a weight heavy enough to create resistance, but not so heavy that it forces you to shift your posture. Feet are shoulder-width apart, core muscles engaged, and shoulder blades are pulled down and back. Either simply hold the weight while standing in place or walk forward while maintaining good posture. Switch the weight to your other hand and repeat.

CO 3: Bird Dog

Purpose: The Bird Dog is an exercise that improves balance and stability, along with strengthening primarily your core and hips (glutes). It also encourages a neutral spine by recruiting back muscles for control as you lift and lower your leg.

How to: You will work opposite arm and leg. As you lift your leg behind you, engage your glute (butt), only lifting as high as you can without arching your back, and reach and lift the opposite arm. If you don't feel like you are doing this right, try poking yourself in the butt of the lifting leg and making that muscle tense.

How to Bird Dog (Standing): Stand facing a wall with your hands at shoulder height, supporting your body with a slight lean toward the wall. You will work the opposite hand and leg. As you slide your right hand up the wall, lift your left leg behind you, keeping your leg straight. Pull in your belly and exhale as you extend your arm and leg. Inhale as you return, then switch to the other side.

How to Bird Dog (Tabletop Position): In Tabletop position (on hands and knees with a flat back), extend one arm without shifting your hips. Next, extend the opposite leg without shifting your hips. Once you've mastered this, lift and extend (reach!) opposite arm and leg without shifting your hips. This is definitely a balance move as much as a core move. Hold, return to tabletop.

Alternate with the other side. When you can do this for both combos of arm/leg, try the bird dog with crunch.

How to Bird Dog (Tabletop with Crunch): After you extend and reach your arm and opposite leg, bring your knee and elbow together under your belly for a crunch. Tighten your abdominal muscles as you do this: pull your belly in like you are zipping up a tight pair of pants.

PILLAR #2 MOVE MORE: RIDE A BIKE THE RIGHT WAY

The focus on cycling, instead of swimming and rowing, is because I believe it to be the very best tool for your knees. You can do it on a stationary bike or ride outdoors. You can look at riding a bike as a joy, as great exercise, or simply as the tool you need to help maintain the health of your knees. Of course, I hope you'll come to love it as I do and appreciate all three factors of why cycling is so good for your knees.

According to Dr. Joseph Garry,[29] "The more the (knee) joint moves through its full range of motion, the more synovial fluid is produced." The continuous motion of bicycling is very helpful for this process of producing more synovial fluid, plus, it is easy on the knees since it is no weight-bearing, no impact, and no lateral movement. To ride most bikes, you need to be able to flex your knee by approximately 110 degrees. This pedaling action and bending of your knee without impact is what is so good for your knee joint. This helps with making your joint's synovial fluid healthier, thicker, and more able to do its job of lubrication and nourishment. Motion is Lotion!

Your bike can be your knees' best friend, as long as it is set up the right way, and you follow basic rules about how fast and how hard to pedal.

I recommend that you start by using an indoor stationary bike as your training tool for knee health because you can control all factors of your ride. No wind, no stoplights, no potholes, no dogs

---

29 Blog.ArthritisFoundation.com, 2018. "Living with Arthritis." Accessed February 15, 2020.
    http://blog.arthritis.org/living-with-arthritis/biking-exercise-for-arthritis/

chasing you, and you don't fall over. You can control your effort when you are working hard and when you are recovering. You can control the length of time you are on your bike because you are not traveling anywhere. You can focus on very specific training techniques and control how much resistance you add, instead of outside, where the terrain controls your effort.

That said, I am an avid outdoor cyclist and love riding my mountain bike, road bike, touring bike, and one-speed pink grocery-getter named Louellen. Like me, you can use the techniques you practice indoor every time that you ride outdoors. This will make you a stronger cyclist and more aware of how you are cycling to protect your knees.

When you are cycling, you are primarily using your leg muscles. The downstroke (pushing down on the pedal) uses your gluteus maximus (big butt muscle) and quadriceps (front of 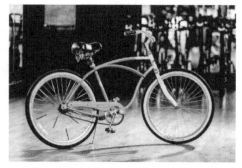 thigh). On the upstroke, when your feet are attached to the pedals (with toe cages or shoes with cleats and clipless pedals), you engage the hamstrings (back of thigh) and hip flexor muscles as you lift the pedal. I recommend using toe cages or clipless pedals so you can effectively engage more muscles throughout your pedal stroke.

BUT WAIT! Don't just hop on your bike! There is a right way and a wrong way to ride.

BIKE FIT IS KEY

There is a specific way to set up your bike to protect your knees. Cycling is a repetitive motion activity that takes your knee through a bending range of about 25 degrees to 110 degrees for every pedal stroke. If you are pedaling at 85 rotations per minute for 30 minutes, that's 2,550 rotations pedaled for each knee! That is why it is critical to set up your bike optimally for your body.

WHAT YOU WANT IN AN INDOOR BIKE

Where do you find an indoor bike? Options are to use one at your local gym or have one at home. If you already own an outdoor bike, it may be possible to mount it on a stand ("trainer") that will turn it into a stationary bike.

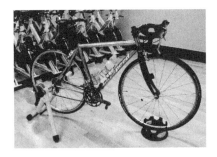

Otherwise, stationary bikes come in two general classifications: upright or recumbent. Upright bikes position the pedals below the seat and are in the style you typically ride outside. Recumbent bikes generally have a chair-like seat with the pedals in front of your seat rather than below it.

I prefer using an upright bike, but it is possible to use a recumbent. Both are great for your knees, and it becomes a matter of preference for body position or availability. As far as I know, recumbent bikes are not yet available as a "spinning style" bike.

"Club Bike" vs. "Spinning Style" Bike

A club bike is a stationary bike with pre-set programs and usually a monitor to display your progress. If you choose a program, the bike automatically adjusts how hard or how easy it is to pedal. Most club bikes will allow you to select a "manual" program so you can adjust the tension. Indoor recumbent bikes are typically "club" bikes with programs. Upright bikes can either be "club" bikes or "spinning style." If you are purchasing a "club" style bike for home use, make sure that you can manually adjust the tension and that the monitor gives you RPM readout (more on that, below).

Spinning style bikes usually have manual adjustments only so that you are always in control of how hard you are working.

For either style of bike, you will want a monitor readout that includes how fast you are pedaling, or RPM (rotations per minute). As you will see later in this chapter, RPM plays a key role in how to ride to protect your knees.

Four Adjustable Points

Ideally, your indoor bike should be adjustable in four locations: Seat height, seat fore/aft (moving seat toward or away from the handlebars), handlebar height, and handlebar fore/aft (moving handlebar toward or away from the seat). I would not recommend any upright indoor bike that does not have all four of these adjustment points.

The bike fit guidelines, below, are designed for an upright bike.

With a recumbent bike, the only adjustment that you can usually make is the position of the seat. Follow the same guideline for seat height for foot position and leg extension (under-seat height).

Bike Fit Step #1: Foot Position

Place the ball of your foot on the center of the pedal. The ball of your foot is the padded part of your foot between your toes and your arch.

If your bike pedals have toe cages, you may not need to push the toe of your shoe to the very end of the toe cage. Toe cages are designed to accommodate a variety of sizes of shoes. No matter your shoe size, center the ball of your foot on the pedal, and your toes may, or may not, reach the end of the toe cage. Tighten the strap of the toe cage so that your foot is snuggly held to the pedal.

What shoes should you wear? For starters, always wear shoes! I learned that lesson the hard way when I was six years old. For cycling, a stiffer soled athletic shoe is better than a really flexible sole, such as a "barefoot" style shoe. There 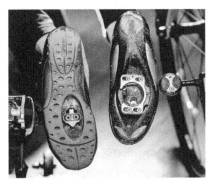 are shoes specially designed for cycling that have a very stiff sole. This helps to support your foot better and reduces the amount of energy lost between the movement of flexing your foot and the pedal. The stiffer the sole, the more power you transfer to the pedal. With a cycling shoe and cleat with "clipless" pedals, instead of using the toe cage to strap your foot to the pedal, you attach with your shoe cleat locking onto the pedal.

Bike Fit Step #2: Seat Height

The goal of adjusting your seat height is to have a 25-35-degree bend in your knee when the pedal is the farthest away from the seat. A 25-35 degree bend in your knee is roughly the bend you would have if you were sitting on the ground with legs extended in front of you, and you placed your fist under your knee; it's a slight bend.

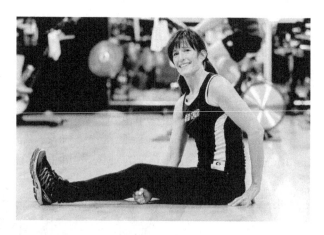

A seat that is too high will cause your knee to be too straight (hyperextension) and may cause pain at the back of your knee or in your low back because you have to rock your hips to stay in contact with the pedals. A seat too low forces a greater knee angle at the top of the pedal stroke, which puts pressure on the patella and quadricep tendon, and can result in pain just above your knee.

Your first guess at adjusting your seat height is to find a starting position, then adjust from there. To find the starting position, stand near your bike seat and lift one leg like you are going to march. Place your thumb in the crease of the fold at your hip and feel around for your front hip bone. While your thumb is on the hip bone, lower your leg and extend your hand out flat. Adjust your seat height to fit just underneath your hand.

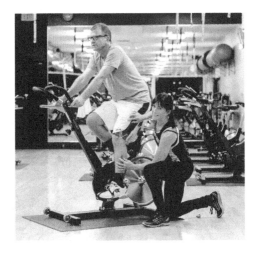

Once you are on your bike, you can double-check the seat height by either measuring your knee bend with a goniometer (which you may not have) or use a simple test. When your pedal is farthest from your seat (at about 5 o'clock if the top of the pedal stroke was "noon"), take the ball of your foot off the pedal and put your heel on the pedal. With your heel on the pedal, your knee should be straight. If it is still bent, your seat needs to be raised. If you had to shift your hips to reach the pedal with your heel, then your seat is too high and should be lowered a bit.

Bike Fit Step #3: Knee Over Pedal
It should be possible to adjust the position of your bike seat closer to or farther from the handlebars. The most important part of the location of your saddle fore or aft is its relationship to where the pedals connect to the bike. On your body, we measure the position of your knee relative to the ball of your foot on the center of the pedal.

First, make sure the ball of your foot is on the center of the pedal while you are sitting on your bike seat. Bring your feet and pedals to the half-way down point, so your pedals are parallel with the floor (this is the 3 o'clock and 9 o'clock position if "noon" is at the top of the pedal and 6 o'clock is at the very bottom.)

When you are in the cycling position, with your hands on the handlebars, look down at your forward foot in the 3 o'clock position. You should be able to see the front part of your foot, from the ball of your foot to the toe of your shoe.

If you see more of your foot (like all the way to your laces), your seat is too far back. This isn't too risky for your knees, but you won't get as much power into the pedals and may feel discomfort in your low back.

If you can't see from the ball of your foot to your toes because your knee is in the way, your seat is too close to your handlebars. It needs to be adjusted back. This is riskier for your knees because you will put more force into your knee joint, and you may feel pain in front of your knee.

Bike Fit Step #4: Handlebar Position

For an indoor bike, comfort is the rule for handlebar height and fore/aft. There is no need to position the handlebars below seat height since you don't need to make an aerodynamic position. Look for a 20-45 degree lean forward for your torso from your hips. Your adjustment goal is to feel about 60-70% of your bodyweight in your saddle and 30-40% of your body weight on your handlebars. In general, you want about an 80-90-degree angle from torso to arm with your hands on the handlebars. A reach farther than that will put too much stress in your shoulders and may cause you pain.

Many people ask me if it is necessary to lean forward to reach the handlebars. The benefit of the forward lean is that it makes it easier to position your sit bones on the saddle. This should be more comfortable overall, and the greater the lean, the deeper the angle at your hips. This deeper angle gives you more potential to use your gluteus maximus while you are pedaling and will engage your core muscles more to help support the position.

Body Position and Comfort

The first thing you will probably think about while riding a bike is your butt. Yes, it does take a little time for your body to get used to the bike seat-butt interface, but with consistency and time (two to four weeks), you won't think about your bottom quite so much.

Your Bottom on the Saddle

Here is the secret to a happy tush on a bike seat: place the pressure of the saddle on your sit bones at the widest part of the seat. To do this, do not tip forward with your hips (which puts painful pressure on your pubic bone area and the soft tissues "down there") and instead, push your sit bones into the back of the saddle where there is the most padding on your hiney and your saddle. You'll then bend forward at your waist to reach the handlebars. Try this first by sitting up straight (let go of the handlebars) and rock your hips forward and backward. Find the place where you feel the pressure on your sit bones and maintain that feeling and pressure as you reach your hands toward the handlebars. It's like a Pilates "C-curl" or a hip tuck.

What shorts should you wear? Snug-fitting bottoms will be better than a loose pair of shorts because they won't bind up in your crotch and rub you the wrong way. Even better are bike shorts with a "pad" (called a chamois or "shammy"). This pad does two things: increases comfort and wicks sweat away. And, by the way, bike shorts are made to be worn without underwear so the sweat-wicking can happen, and there is no stress from underwear elastic binding up.

Your Feet: Remember to place the ball of your foot, not the arch of your foot on the pedal.

Your Back: Keep a fairly flat back as you lean forward

Your Shoulders-Elbows-Wrists-Hands: This kinetic chain should be relaxed. Any tension along the way can cause hands to go numb or create tension in your neck.

Shoulders: take a big breath in and raise your shoulders right up to your ears, and as you exhale, totally relax your shoulders. This relaxed state is where you want your shoulders while you ride.

Elbows: Keep a soft bend in your elbows. Stick-straight arms can cause tension in shoulders and neck or make your hands go numb. Let your core muscles hold you up, not straight arms.

Wrists: As you hang onto the handlebars, do not bend your wrists. This puts a lot of pressure on the radial nerve that comes from your arm to your hand and may make your fingers go numb. Keep a long line from your forearm to your wrist and your wrists straight as you hold the handlebars.

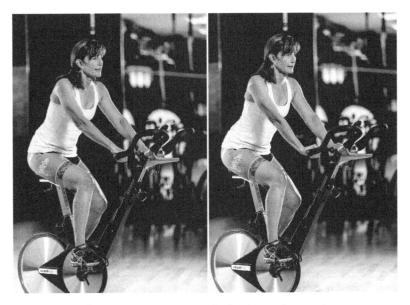

Left picture: correct wrists. Right picture: bent wrists

Hands: No need to have a death grip on the handlebars! When on an indoor bike, you do not need to steer. Use a light grip with the weight on the thickest pad on the palm of your hand (the "heel" of your hand) near the base of your thumb.

HOW FAST AND HOW HARD TO PEDAL?
There is more to taking care of your knees on a bike than just spinning your wheels.

Pedal Dynamics
In order to get the biggest benefit from your time on the bike, I recommend that you attach your feet to your pedals either with toe cages or clipless pedals and wearing shoes with bike cleats in the bottom. These attachments will give you the chance to engage more leg muscles throughout the pedal stroke.

We break the pedal stroke into four parts: downstroke (pushing down), bottom stroke (pulling the pedal back), upstroke (lifting up), and top stroke (kicking over the top). To practice this, you will pedal all the way around but emphasize one of the four parts at a time. If you are on a stationary bike, you can even close your eyes to focus deeper on the sensation of what you are feeling as you are pedaling.

Downstroke

Pushing down on the pedals is where you get the most power. This is initiated with your gluteus maximus and continued with your quadriceps.

Main Muscles: Butt (gluteus maximus) and thigh (quadriceps).

What You Should Feel: Pressure on the ball of your foot as you push against the pedal.

Bottom Stroke

Pull back on the pedal like you are trying to scrape mud off the bottom of your shoe, or you are a bull about to charge.

Main Muscles: Calf, front of shin, and some back of thigh (hamstrings).

What You Should Feel: Pressure at the back of your heel as it pulls against your shoe as you pull your foot back.

Upstroke

Lift up on the pedal as if you are trying to kick your butt with your heel, but keep your foot fairly level to the ground. This is a

great move to use as training if you want to become more powerful when riding hills on your bike outside.

Main Muscles: Hamstrings, hip flexors, and side leg (tensor fascia
latae for hip abduction).

What you should feel: The top of your foot lift against the top
of your shoe while you keep your foot relatively parallel to the
ground (0-25-degree heel lift).

Top stroke
Kick over the top of the pedal stroke forcefully like you are kicking a ball with the toe of each foot.

Main Muscles: Quadriceps, gluteus maximus, and tensor fascia latae.

What You Should Feel: Like you are shooting your foot forward.
You may notice your pedal speed increases as you focus on the
top stroke because you just got a little more efficient.

THE SECRETS TO PEDAL SPEED, RESISTANCE, AND PERCEIVED EFFORT
We recommend that you follow the Healthy Knee Pedal Speed
Rule: 60-110 rotations per minute (RPM). Start with light tension
so you can comfortably pedal in this range. 60 RPM is one pedal
revolution per second. If your bike does not have a monitor that
displays RPM, you can count it by watching the seconds on a clock.
On the faster pedal speed end of the scale, 110 RPM is almost two
full pedal rotations per second.

Too Slow: Many people tend to pedal slowly with too much resistance, and that puts more torque force in your knee joint on every push of the pedals. I want you to start practicing the parts of the pedal stroke and adjusting your tension so you can pedal a minimum of 60 RPM. Then, eventually, I hope 85-95 RPM will become your comfort zone for base general riding and reserve the 60-70 RPM for "hills."

Too Fast: On the other hand, spinning as fast as you can with little tension is not good either. Indoor cycling bikes usually have a weighted flywheel that, once it gets going, can carry your feet if you are not in control. This puts your knees at risk! If you find you are pedaling along and your hips start bumping in the saddle, this shows you are not in control of the pedals, and they are controlling you. To correct for this, either slow your pedal speed or add more tension. You'll stop hopping around and regain control.

How much resistance (tension) should you add? Well, that all depends on how hard you want to work. At first, it is better to use light tension so you can get the hang of the four parts of the pedal stroke and reduce the risk of too much force through the knee joint.

Healthy Knees Coach uses 5 Zones of Perceived Exertion:
- Zone 1 = Easy effort, breathing easy
- Zone 2 = Moderate effort working in your comfort zone, could still carry on a conversation
- Zone 3 = Hard effort, outside your comfort zone and breathing is elevated, can have short conversation

- Zone 4 = Very hard effort, sustainable for a short time, breathing hard, conversation reduced to a few words
- Zone 5 = All out maximum effort sustainable for only 10-15 seconds, breathing is more like panting, conversation more like a grunt

It is most important to focus on Zones 1, 2, and 3 in the beginning. Don't worry about Zones 4 and 5; you won't get to them for some time in your training. The key is to know what RPM and zone you want to be in and how to adjust your tension to achieve that zone.

RIDE GUIDE

To start, I recommend that you ride two to three times per week to see and feel a change with your knees. Something is better than nothing! If you cannot do the recommended time, just do what you can and work up to more.

Here are three example rides to get you started. Each ride can be repeated as many times as you want until you feel comfortable. I recommend that you repeat each ride at least twice in a week (e.g., use Ride #1 two times in your first week).

Healthy Knees Total Knee Replacement RIDE #1: Introducing Pedal Stroke					24 Min Total
RIDE Time	Interval Time	Focus	Cue	RPM	ZONE
0–4	4:00	Warm Up	Easy spin. Add enough tension so you feel you are pushing against something	60+	1
4–12	8:00	Pedal Stroke	4X Practice the parts of pedal stroke for 0:30 each: Downstroke, Bottom stroke, Upstroke, Top stroke	60–90	2
12–14	2:00	Recovery	Easy Pedal	60+	1
14–18	4:00	Pedal Stroke	2X 0:30 on each pedal Stroke Downstroke, Bottom stroke, Upstroke, Top stroke	60–90	2
18–19	1:00	Perfect Pedal Stroke	Blend all 4 pedal stroke parts together: pedal like you are trying to make a bigger circle than your pedals will allow.	70–90	2
19–24	5:00	Cool down	Easy spin	60+	1

Healthy Knees Total Knee Replacement RIDE #2: Pedal Speed Practice					24 Min Total
RIDE Time	Interval Time	Focus	Cue	RPM	ZONE
0-5	5:00	Warm Up	Easy spin. Add enough tension, so you feel you are pushing against something	60+	1
5-10	5:00	Pedal Stroke Practice each part: Downstroke, Bottom stroke, Upstroke, Top stroke	2X for 0:30 each: 1X ea for 0:15 each	70-90	2
10-11	1:00	Perfect Pedal Stroke	Use force all the way around to feel like pedaling a circle bigger than pedals allow	70-90	2
11-13	2:00	Recovery	Easy Pedal	70=	1
13-16:30	3:30	Pedal Speed	Practice each RPM for 0:30 each: Reduce resistance if it gets too hard as you go faster.	60-65-70-75-80-85-90	2
16:30-17:30	1:00	Recovery	Easy Pedal	70+	1
17:30-21	3:30	Pedal Speed	Practice each RPM for 0:30 each: Reduce resistance if it gets too hard as you go faster.	60-65-70-75-80-85-90	2
21-26	5:00	Cool Down	Easy spin	60+	1

Healthy Knees Total Knee Replacement RIDE #3: Introducing Resistance					28 Min Total
RIDE Time	Interval Time	Focus	Cue	RPM	ZONE
0–5	5:00	Warm Up	Easy spin. Add enough tension, so you feel you are pushing against something	60+	1
5–10	5:00	Pedal Stroke Practice each part: Downstroke, Bottom stroke, Upstroke, Top stroke	2X for 0:30 each: 1X for 0:15 each	70–90	1–2
10–11	1:00	Perfect Pedal Stroke	Use force all the way around to feel like you are pedaling a circle bigger than pedals allow.	70–90	2
11–12	1:00	Easy Pedal	Light & Easy	60+	1
12–15:30	3:30	Pedal Speed	Practice each RPM for 0:30 each: Reduce resistance if it gets too hard as you go faster.	60–65–70–75–80–85–90	2
15:30–17	1:30	Easy Pedal	Light & Easy	60+	1

| Healthy Knees Total Knee Replacement RIDE #3: Introducing Resistance | | | | | 28 Min Total |
RIDE Time	Interval Time	Focus	Cue	RPM	ZONE
17-19	2:00	Resistance Drills	Hold 70 RPM 0:60 Easy (Zone 1) 0:30 Moderate (Zone 2) 0:30 Hard (Zone 3)	70	1-2-3
19-21	2:00	Resistance Drills	Hold 75 RPM 0:60 Easy (Zone 1) 0:30 Moderate (Zone 2) 0:30 Hard (Zone 3)	75	1-2-3
21-23	2:00	Resistance Drills	Hold 80 RPM 0:60 Easy (Zone 1) 0:30 Moderate (Zone 2) 0:30 Hard (Zone 3)	80	1-2-3
23-28	5:00	Cool Down	Easy spin	60+	1

If you want more than just these three rides, I hope you will check out our Healthy Knees Formula online program, which includes a guided video weekly program to help you keep advancing and more help to make sure you are doing it right. www.healthykneesformula.com

PILLAR #3 GET FLEXIBLE: PRACTICE STRETCH AND RELEASE TECHNIQUES

Regular stretching helps prepare your muscles for the work to come and to recover from the work you just completed. Stretching will help you improve the range of motion of your knees (and other joints) and help improve your flexibility. All of the stretches described below should be done daily.

STRETCH TECHNIQUES

We have divided stretches into three distinct groups:

1. Dynamic Stretches
2. Static Stretches
3. Release Techniques

DYNAMIC STRETCHES

Dynamic stretching means you repeat controlled movement in and out of the stretch position. It is an important part of warming up your muscles for the work ahead. Warm-up is a very important part of your transition from a resting state to one that is ready for action. During your warm-up, your body will direct more blood to your working muscles.

When we focus on your knees, we will perform warm-ups for your hips and knees.

- Knee ROM and Hold
- Pigeon Rocking
- Hip Hurdles and Swivel

Knee ROM and Hold

Purpose: This passive range-of-motion (ROM) drill is meant to help provide more low level and low impact knee flexion volume. It will help promote better knee flexion ranges, gradually address any fear, and familiarize you with the sensation of deep knee bends.

How to (Standing): Place your foot on a chair and rock into the knee bend until you feel pressure, but no pain. Rock 10X on each leg. On the last rock, hold the stretch at least 30 seconds and up to 2 minutes (as long as it doesn't cause pain).

How to (in Tabletop Position): While on your hands and knees (you can use a foam pad for your knees if you want), rock forward to decrease the bend in your knee and rock backward to increase the knee bend so that you feel pressure, but no pain. Repeat 10X, and on the last one, hold the deepest knee bend you can for 30 seconds up to 2 minutes.

Pigeon Rocking

Purpose: This is a mobility drill designed to target the entire hip and its surrounding muscles, as well as the hip capsule itself. The goal is to open up both internal and external rotation at the hip, allowing for easier movement.

How to: Starting on all fours, straighten one leg as far as you can straight behind you. Then, swivel the other leg under your body to somewhere between a 45- and 90-degree angle compared to your midline. From here, take the straight leg, and reach it across your body, so you are creating more tension in the bent leg hip. Slowly rock your weight backward and bend the straight leg knee to drop it to the floor. You should feel a stretch increase in the opposite hip. Slowly rock back and forth, bending and straightening the knee to allow you to sink deeper and deeper into the stretch.

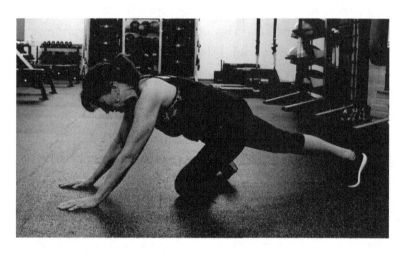

Hip Hurdles and Swivel

Purpose: This drill warms up your hip joint and works on mobility. We like this move because it helps make your hips feel smoother in their action.

How to: Stand tall with your hands on your hips. Lift your right knee and leg as if you are going to step over a fence or a hurdle. Rotate your leg to the right, keeping your knee high. Set your foot on the ground. Your feet should now make a 90-degree angle, with your left foot pointing forward and your right foot pointing to the right. Reverse the move by lifting your leg back up and over the imaginary hurdle. Place your foot back on the ground with both feet pointing forward. Repeat on the left leg.

After you have completed ten on each leg, it's time to swivel! Stand with your feet about hip width apart, toes forward, and hands on hips. Start thinking "Hula" and make big clockwise circles 10X with your hips, then repeat in the reverse direction.

STATIC STRETCHES

Static Stretching means you achieve and hold the stretch position. The purpose of static stretching is to elongate muscle fibers to help improve flexibility and reduce the risk of injury. To have the best results, static stretching can be done daily after you have warmed up or, better yet, at the end of your exercise activity as part of your cool down.

Hold each stretch from 30 seconds to two minutes. Use deep breathing as part of your stretching technique where on each exhale, you try to relax and stretch a little deeper.

- Calf
- Hamstring
- Side Leg Stretch
- Figure 4 Hip
- Quadriceps
- Half-Kneeling Hip Flexor

Calf Stretch

Purpose: The calf stretch focuses on your two calf muscles, the gastrocnemius and soleus, which merge into the Achilles tendon.

How to: This two-part stretch can be done standing (unassisted) or assisted by placing your hands on a wall at about shoulder height and leaning toward the wall. Take a large step backward with one foot. With both feet pointing forward (this is key to getting the stretch), keep your weight on your bent front leg. Press the heel of your back leg toward the floor for a calf stretch with a straight leg and hold. Then add the second stretch by slightly bending the knee of your back leg and continue pressing your heel to the ground. Bending your knee shifts the stretch toward your Achilles tendon.

Hamstring Stretch

Purpose: Three muscles make up your hamstrings. They all originate on your "sit bones" pelvic bone. The semimembranosus and semitendinosus attach on the medial side of your knee to the tibia. The bicep femoris actually has two origins, one on the pelvis and one on the femur. The whole bicep femoris muscle attaches to the head of the fibula. Many people have tight hamstrings from constantly sitting with knees bent (thus shortening the hamstring group). Tight hamstrings can make your knees sore and even pull on your pelvis and create an unwanted pelvic tilt. The hamstring stretch will help relieve hamstring tension.

How to: While standing, step one foot forward with a straight leg. Transfer your weight to your back leg with knee slightly bent. With a flat back and hands resting on your thighs, hinge forward at your hips. Take in a deep breath. As you exhale, raise your forward toe off the ground and stretch a little deeper. Keeping your back flat is the key to this stretch. Step back to standing and repeat on the other side.

Side Leg Stretch

Purpose: This move helps stretch the muscles associated with the Iliotibial Band (ITB), which include your tensor fasciae latae and gluteus maximus muscles, both at your hip. The IT Band itself is a very thick sheath of fascia (connective tissue) that runs the length of the outside of your leg from hip to knee. The ITB works to stabilize the hip during walking and acts as a spring to aid in running.[30] You may notice a difference in how far you can reach on each side for this one.

How to: While standing, cross your left foot in front of your right so that your feet are side-by-side. Now press your hands together. Hinge at your hips and reach with hands toward the instep of your back (right) foot. Hold, then return to standing. Complete the stretch on the other side.

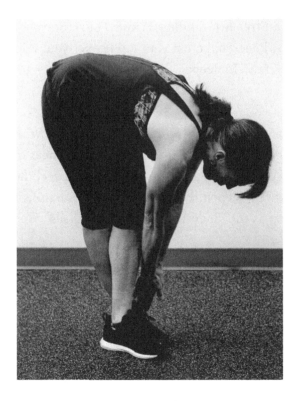

---

30 The Harvard Gazette, 2015. "Understanding the IT Band." Accessed January 5, 2020. https://news.harvard.edu/gazette/story/2015/08/understanding-the-it-band/

Figure 4 Hip Stretch

Purpose: The figure-four stretch can be done standing or lying down. Do the one that feels the best for you and repeat on each leg. You will feel this stretch in the outside of your hip.

How to Hip Stretch (Figure Four with Chair Assist): Shift your weight to your left leg and place your right foot on a chair. Let the right knee rotate away from your midline toward the floor. To deepen the stretch, press on your thigh (not your knee).

How to Hip Stretch (Standing Figure Four): Start with a slight bend in your knees and cross your ankle over your opposite thigh above your knee. To deepen the stretch, press on your thigh (not your knee).

How to Hip Stretch (Figure Four on the Floor): Lie with your back on the floor and cross your legs, bringing your knees toward your chest. Hug your knees, and you should feel a nice deep stretch in your butt. To deepen the stretch, press your shins toward the floor, as long as this does not irritate your knees.

How to Hip Stretch (Figure Four Reach Through): To make the floor stretch even deeper, cross your right ankle over your left thigh, just above your knee. Clasp your hands behind your left thigh to gently pull your leg closer to your chest.

Quadriceps Stretch

Purpose: The basic movement is to bend at the knee, bringing your heel toward your butt. Depending on your knee range of motion, you may need help with this one.

As you perform the stretch, keep your knees side by side and focus on standing tall with your hips pressed forward and shoulders back.

How to Quad Stretch (Assist with a Chair): Standing in front of a chair like you are going to sit down, raise one leg behind you and rest the top of your foot on the chair with your knee pointing toward the floor. You might want to be near a wall for balance and may need to bend the supporting leg to deepen the stretch.

How to Quad Stretch (Assist with a Towel): Start standing and bend over to wrap a small towel around one ankle. Hold the towel near your ankle with the same side hand. As you return to standing, lift your towel-ankle toward your butt behind you.

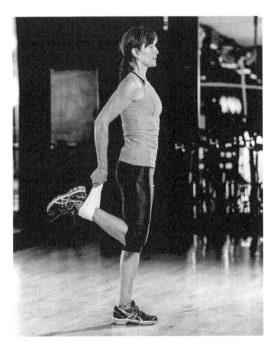

How to Quad Stretch (No Assist): This is only for you if you have the ability to fully flex your knee. If you have limited range of motion, use one of the assists.

While standing, bring your heel toward your butt and grab onto your ankle. Your knees should be side by side and body erect. If you go through any gymnastics to do this or your knee is sticking out to the side, or if you are side bending one way or the other, *don't!* This poor alignment could strain your back. Use one of the assists, above.

Half-Kneeling Hip Flexor Stretch

Purpose: This passive stretch is designed to provide a stretch to the hip flexor (iliopsoas) muscle group.

How to Hip Flexor Stretch (Standing): Standing with feet hip-width apart, raise both arms overhead and touch hands together. While you look up at your hands, press your hips forward and tilt backward (but do not "arch" your back). Hold for a count of 5.

How to Hip Flexor Stretch (Half Kneeling): For a deeper stretch than you can get in the standing position, place the foam pad or pillow beneath the right knee as you get into a half-kneeling position with your right knee down and left foot on the floor in front of you. The left hip and leg should be flexed to 90 degrees. Next, fully raise your right arm overhead like you are trying to reach the ceiling. Squeeze your right butt (glute) and slowly shift your torso forward, allowing the right hip to extend. You should feel the stretch through the front of your right hip. To deepen the stretch, tuck your hips (posterior pelvic tilt).

RELEASE TECHNIQUES

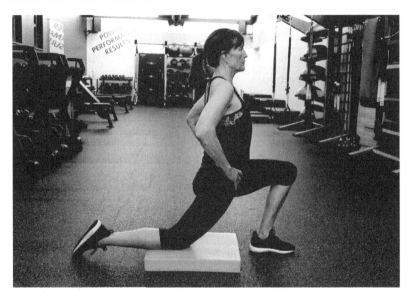

Piriformis Release

The Piriformis is a muscle deep in your butt that originates at the sacrum (near your tail bone) and attaches to the side knob (greater trochanter) near the top of the femur. It helps to lift and rotate your leg away from the midline. The piriformis can irritate the nearby sciatic nerve and cause "Piriformis Syndrome" with pain originating in the buttocks and radiating down the leg. Of course, if you have sciatic nerve pain, please see your doctor! Sciatic pain can also be caused by compression in the spine.[31]

Purpose: This trigger point method places pressure on a sensitive or sore spot in a muscle so that when the pressure is released,

---

31 National Academy of Sports Medicine, 2018. "Piriformis: Is it Really Tight? Really?" Accessed December 28, 2019. https://blog.nasm.org/fitness/piriformis-is-it-really-tight-really/

circulation increases, and the muscle relaxes. I include this release because, to me, it feels good, and I feel like it helps my butt and my legs stay a little more relaxed. Does it actually help relax the muscle? I don't know, but you will feel the difference as soon as you complete the move.

How to: Use the Hero Rollga ball or hard ball, such as a lacrosse ball or a tennis ball. While sitting on the floor with your legs extended straight in front of you, take the ball and pretend you are slipping it into your back right pocket. Gently "sit" on the ball and position it on the spot that feels the most tender. Now bend and straighten your right leg four times, sliding your foot toward your butt then back to straight leg. Next, with your right knee bent and foot on the ground, let your knee dip toward your left leg four times. Then, let your knee lower toward the floor away from your left leg, four times. Finally, straighten your leg, sit up tall, and—this is where the magic happens—remove the ball and feel the "cave" in your butt. NICE! Make sure and repeat this release on your left side too.

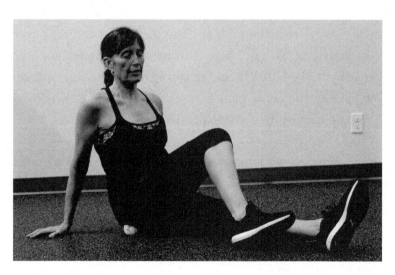

Myofascial Release

The current literature measuring the effects of self-myofascial release is still emerging. Fascia is a web of connective tissue that covers every internal structure of the body. We've included foam rolling in this book because I've personally had so much relief from performing regular rolling on my own legs. It is definitely worth a try and, with time, if it makes you feel better, great! Foam rolling can be done either pre- or post-exercise.

Purpose: Foam rolling places pressure on your skin, fascia, and underlying muscle with the idea that the pressure stretches fascial tissue and increases blood flow once the pressure is released. Foam rolling can be done as a warm-up to increase circulation before exercise. It can also be done post-exercise as some studies have shown that foam rolling may be beneficial in relieving muscle soreness and improving passive and dynamic range of motion[32] [33]

I like to foam roll before I exercise when I am going to focus on range of motion and after exercise, especially after long bike rides where my legs feel tired.

How to: There are many techniques to rolling, but the one I find most beneficial is to lie on the roller and start at the distal end of the muscle group (the point farther away from your core). Roll up about 4 inches, back 2 inches, up 4 inches, and back 2 inches,

---

32 Frontiers in Physiology, 2019. "A Meta-Analysis of the Effects of Foam Rolling on Performance and Recovery." Accessed January 5, 2020. https://www.ncbi.nlm.nih.gov/pmc/articles/PMC6465761/

33 Medicine and Science in Sports and Exercise, 2014. "Foam Rolling as a Recovery Tool after an Intense Bout of Physical Activity." Accessed January 5, 2020. https://journals.lww.com/acsm-msse/Fulltext/2014/01000/Foam_Rolling_as_a_Recovery_Tool_after_an_Intense.19.aspx.

slowly inch-worming up your leg; then reverse direction and roll, using the same method back to your starting point. Pay special attention to your quadriceps, Iliotibial band (IT Band, the side of your leg), hamstring, and calf.

If you are unable to maneuver your body onto the floor to use a foam roller (this does require a certain amount of core strength), you can try sitting in a chair with your leg relaxed and the same technique (4 inches up, 2 inches back) with an old fashioned rolling pin to roll your quads and IT band.

PILLAR #4 EAT SMARTER: PREPARE FOR AND RECOVER FROM SURGERY FASTER WITH THE RIGHT NUTRITION
By Dr. Stephen Black

It is a well-known fact that proper nutrition is essential in the performance of and recovery from sports and recreational activities. This same premise applies to your preparation for your surgery. Science-focused evidence points to the appropriate type, amount, and timing of intake of food, fluids, and dietary supplement to promote optimal health. The one-size-fits-all approach could lead to delayed recovery, including when surgery is indicated.

Nutrition goals and requirements are not static. Nutrition related to preparing for and recovering from surgery should target specific strategies that reduce fatigue and maintain optimal cellular performance. These strategies will account for maximizing results, reducing disease risk, and improving healing. As was discussed previously, optimizing body weight is essential for the longevity of your TKR. It also affects immune system integrity, hormonal balance, and injury prevention. Preparing for surgery is a great time to clean up your eating habits both for weight loss (if needed) and cellular preparation.

NUTRITION BASICS

Appropriate energy intake is the cornerstone to support optimal body function. First, a mini nutrition lesson. Nutrients are divided into two categories: Macronutrients and Micronutrients.

Macronutrients

Macronutrients are what your body needs in large amounts and make up the bulk of the nutrition in foods: all foods are either carbohydrates, proteins, fats, or a combination. These three macronutrients serve as the building blocks for muscles, brain function, and tissues (maintenance, recovery, and repair).

Carbohydrates		Proteins		Fats
Berries				
Bran				
Bread		Bison	Bacon	
Corn		Buffalo		
Couscous	Beans	Chicken	Chia Seeds	Avocado
Cream of Wheat		Egg Whites		
English Muffins	Most Yogurts	Fish	Cottage Cheese	Egg Yolks
Fruits		Lean Beef		
Oats	Peas	Low/Non-fat	Duck	Flaxseed
Pancakes		Cottage Cheese		
Pasta	Quinoa	Low/Non-fat	Eggs	Nut Butters
Potatoes		Greek Yogurt		
Pumpkin	Skim Milk	Turkey	Salmon	Nuts
Rice		Turkey Bacon		
Squash	Sprouted Grains	Whey Protein	Whole Fat Milk	Oils
Sugars				
Vegetables			Whole-Fat Yogurt	Olives
Whole Grains				
Whole Wheat				

Carbohydrates

Carbohydrates have received a great deal of attention in sports nutrition and rightfully so. This nutrient plays a critical role in performance and adaptation to training. Carbohydrates offer advantages over fats as a fuel source because they provide a greater yield of energy per volume of oxygen, thus improving exercise efficiency. Carbohydrates are also a key fuel source for the brain and central nervous system along with muscular work. Carbohydrates have four calories per gram.

Depleting carbohydrate stores is associated with fatigue. Have you ever heard of "bonking" or "hitting the wall?" It's like you've suddenly run out of all energy, and your body feels like cement. This happens largely because you've used up your stores of carbohydrates.

Unfortunately, the body stores relatively little carbohydrate and the amount stored and used changes daily based on dietary intake (storage). Even a single session of exercise uses stored carbohydrates to create energy for your muscles.

Here is an example of carbohydrate needs depending on the intensity of activity. The timing of the carbohydrate intake may be manipulated to promote high carb availability for exercise sessions or recovery.

ACTIVITY LEVEL	CARB TARGET for body weight	# Grams for 150 lb person
Light (low intensity)	3-5g/kg or 1.4-2.3g/lb	345 g
Moderate	5-7g/kg or 2.3-3.2g/lb	375–480 g
High (endurance or high intensity 1-3 hr/day)	6-10g/kg or 2.7-4.5g/lb	405–675g
Very High (4-5 hr/day HIIT)	8-12g/kg or 3.6-5.4g/lb	540–810 g

Proteins

Protein is an essential part of every cell in your body. Proteins, when digested, are broken down into their amino acid components that are used by the body in a multitude of ways. A dietary protein is considered "complete" when it contains all essential amino acids. An amino acid is considered "essential" when it must be ingested because it cannot be made in the body.

Proteins help the body not only build muscle, but also break down food, and control cellular processes. Proteins enhance structural changes in tissues such as fascia, tendon, and bone, which is key in recovering from a surgery such as a total knee replacement.

With injury or surgery, elevated protein needs are required for healing and to prevent muscle atrophy. Muscle atrophy, or loss of muscle, often happens during recovery as you are unable to move or exercise in normal ways.

Protein has four calories per gram. Current data suggest that dietary protein intake necessary to support metabolic adaptation, along with tissue and bone repair, generally ranges from 1.8—2.5g/kg/day (0.82-1.13g/lb/day). The higher recommendations are for short periods of highly intensified training, like preparing for and recovering from surgery.

For a 150-pound person, this would equal 123-170 grams of protein per day.

Fat

Fat is a necessary part of a healthy diet that provides energy and keeps our cells healthy. Your own body makes fat from storing excess calories.

Fat has nine calories per gram, double the calories of carbohydrates or protein (four calories per gram). In general, unsaturated fats are better, trans-fats are bad, and saturated fats are somewhere in between. When discussing fats that we eat, you'll hear the terms "unsaturated" and "saturated." This refers to the amount of hydrogen in the molecule, and the type of chemical structure it has: a fat molecule with as many hydrogen atoms as possible is "saturated."

Monounsaturated fats are liquid at room temperature but may solidify when cooled. The lower the temperature needed for solidification, the lesser the degree of saturation. Good sources include extra virgin olive oil, which is cold-pressed and unrefined, peanuts, and avocados in their natural form, along with salmon and other cold-water fish. Peanut oil, avocado oil, olive oil, and unrefined canola oil are examples of culinary oils that are monounsaturated fats.

Polyunsaturated fatty acids and essential fatty acids are cholesterol free. This is good! Examples of foods high in polyunsaturated fats include cold-water fish (salmon, tuna, trout), walnuts, black beans, brussels sprouts, sunflower seeds, and flax seeds. However, polyunsaturated fatty acids in culinary oils, such as safflower, corn, sesame, and soy oils, are unstable when heated and susceptible to oxidation by free radicals (a highly reactive molecule) during storage.[34] When consumed, free radicals can damage DNA, alter cell membranes, and promote cancer.[35] While it's great to eat these fats in our food, you don't want to cook with them, especially at high heat.

Saturated fats are solid at room temperature. Butter, cheese, and cream are high in saturated fat, as are the white fat on meat and meat products and tropical oils. Saturated fats may potentially increase the amount of LDL cholesterol in the blood and are also associated with the development of insulin resistance. These outcomes are typically seen when saturated fat is combined with high glycemic, inflammatory carbohydrates. Saturated fats should be consumed in limited quantities.

Trans-fatty acids or hydrogenated fats are oils that have been artificially saturated with hydrogen to create a solid. The resulting solid fat has a long shelf life, is stable at high temperatures, and is used in commercially prepared foods. Common foods are highly processed commercially baked goods, fried foods, vegetable oils, and margarines. The consumption of trans-fatty acids is shown to negatively affect cholesterol levels and impair metabolic processes in cardiac tissue.[36]

Total fat intake (both saturated and unsaturated fat) should not exceed 20%-35% daily. Most sources recommend we ingest no more

34 Pubmed.gov, 1995. "Free Radicals in Foods." Accessed March 6, 2020. https://www. ncbi.nlm.nih.gov/pubmed/7704185

35 Pharmacognosy Review, 2010. "Free Radicals, Antioxidants and Functional Foods: Impact On Human Health." Accessed February 29, 2020. https://www.ncbi.nlm.nih.gov/pmc/ articles/PMC3249911/.

36 Replace Trans Fat. Accessed March 6, 2020. https://www.who.int/docs/default-source/ documents/replace-transfats/replace-trans-fat-faqs.pdf?Status=Temp&sfvrsn=956d171f_6

than 10% of saturated fat daily. Trans-fatty acids and hydrogenated fats should be avoided.

Fat intake for a 150-pound person would be approximately 33-113 grams per day.

Example Food Sources of Dietary Fats		
Unsaturated Fats	Saturated Fats	Trans Fats
Fish (salmon, tuna, trout)	Beef	Deep Fried Chicken
Olive Oil	Butter	Margarine or Vegetable Shortening
Baked Potatoes	Scalloped Potatoes	French Fries
Almonds, Hazelnuts, Pecans	Ice Cream	Refrigerated dough (biscuits and rolls)

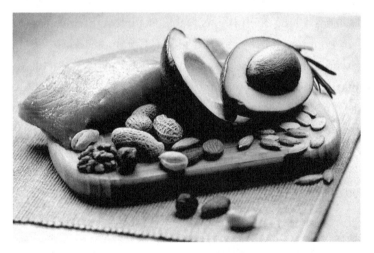

Healthy fats look tasty too [37]

Micronutrients

Micronutrients are individual vitamins and minerals your body needs in smaller amounts. In general, vitamins are needed for energy production, immune function, and blood clotting. They help to keep your skin, gastrointestinal tract, eyes, lungs, and nervous system in good working order. Minerals help our bodies to grow, develop, and stay healthy while keeping our bones, muscles, heart, and brain working properly. Minerals also play a key role in making enzymes and hormones.[38]

Micronutrient & Function	Common Dietary Sources
VITAMINS	
Vitamin A (Retinol) • Essential for normal vision and immune function • Needed for cell growth and development • b-carotene can be converted to vitamin A by the liver as needed	Retinol: beef liver, fortified cereal, eggs, butter, fortified milk b-Carotene: sweet potatoes, pumpkins, carrots, cantaloupes, mangoes, spinach, broccoli, kale, collards, butternut squash
Thiamin (Vitamin B1) • Assists the release of energy from carbohydrates and protein	Fortified cereal, bread, pork, enriched white rice, brown rice, peas, macadamia nuts, sunflower seeds, beans, lentils, cantaloupe
Riboflavin (Vitamin B2) • Assists the release of energy from fat, carbohydrates, and protein • Assists several antioxidant enzymes	Milk, fortified cereal, bread, eggs, almonds, clams, spinach, chicken, beef, asparagus, salmon, cheese, broccoli

---

38 NIB, 2019. "Vitamins and Minerals: What's the Difference and What Are They For?" https://www.nib.com.au/the-checkup/healthy-living/vitamins-and-minerals-whats-the-difference

Micronutrient & Function	Common Dietary Sources
VITAMINS	
Niacin (Vitamin B3) • Assists the release of energy from fat, carbohydrates, and protein	Chicken breast, tuna, turkey, salmon, anchovies, ground beef, liver, peanuts, avocado, brown rice, mushrooms
Pantothenic Acid (Vitamin B5) • Assists the release of energy from fat, carbohydrates, and protein • Assists fat, cholesterol, steroid hormones, and hemoglobin synthesis	Avocados, yogurt, chicken, sweet potatoes, milk, lentils, eggs, peas, mushrooms, fish, broccoli
Vitamin B6 • Supports a wide variety of metabolic reactions • Assists neurotransmitters, hemoglobin, and DNA production • Influences steroid hormone action	Turkey, chicken, fortified cereal, bread, potatoes (with skin), fish, prunes, bananas, hazelnuts, walnuts, pork, beans
Biotin (Vitamin B7) • Assists the release of energy from fat, carbohydrates, and protein • Assists in glucose production	Beef liver, eggs, salmon, avocados, yeast, whole-wheat bread, pork, cheese
Folate (Vitamin B9) • Required for DNA synthesis • Assists red blood cell production • Prevents neural tube defects • Folic acid, found in supplements and fortified food, is more readily absorbed than naturally occurring folate	Folate: beans, lentils, asparagus, spinach, peanuts, peas, corn, chicken, orange juice Folic Acid: enriched rice or products made with enriched flours, such as cereal, pasta, or bread

Micronutrient & Function	Common Dietary Sources

VITAMINS

Vitamin B12
- Assists the release of energy from fat and protein
- Assists hemoglobin and red blood cell production
- Required for nerve function

Clams, mussels, crab meat, salmon, beef, rockfish, milk, cheese, eggs, chicken, turkey, fortified cereal

Vitamin C
- Antioxidant in blood and cells
- Augments functional activity of immune cells
- Assists collagen, carnitine, serotonin, and adrenaline production

Chili peppers, sweet peppers, guavas, kiwifruits, strawberries, oranges, kale, spinach, broccoli, grapefruit, potatoes, tomatoes

Vitamin D
- Maintains calcium and phosphorus balance
- Promotes bone health and immune function
- Influences cell growth and development
- Vitamin D is made from cholesterol in your skin when it is exposed to the sun

Fish (especially salmon, tuna, herring, sardines, and mackerel), eggs, fortified soy milk, fortified orange juice, fortified milk, fortified cereal

Vitamin E
- Antioxidant in cell membranes
- Supports normal nerve function
- Augments functional activity of immune cells

Olive oil, safflower oil, sunflower oil, almonds, hazelnuts, peanuts, spinach, carrots, avocados

Vitamin K
- Assists in blood clotting
- Modifies certain proteins to allow for calcium binding

Kale, chard, parsley, broccoli, spinach, watercress, leaf lettuce, cashews, peas, soybean oil, canola oil, olive oil, mayonnaise, naturally fermented food

Micronutrient & Function	Common Dietary Sources
MINERALS	
Calcium • Structural component of bones and teeth • Required for proper nerve transmission and muscle contraction • Influences blood vessel constriction and dilation and may reduce blood pressure	Milk, yogurt, cheese, tofu (calcium set), fortified beverages, fortified cereal, rhubarb, spinach, almonds, white beans, bok choy, kale, pinto beans, red beans, broccoli
Chromium • Assists insulin action	Broccoli, grape juice, sweet potatoes, orange juice, beef, turkey, chicken, apples (with peel), green beans, tomatoes, bananas
Copper • Assists in energy production and iron utilization • Assists in neurotransmitter synthesis • Maintains integrity of connective tissue • Assists antioxidant enzymes	Beef liver, oysters, crab meat, clams, sunflower seeds, kale, cashews, lentils, beans, mushrooms, cocoa powder, raisins, peanut butter
Fluoride • Structural component of bones and teeth	Fluoridated water, crab meat, beans, black tea, raisins, cereal, fish, fruit juice
Iodine • Component of thyroid hormones	Cod, iodized salt, potatoes (with skin), milk, shrimp, turkey, navy beans, tuna, eggs, seaweed

Micronutrient & Function	Common Dietary Sources
MINERALS	

Iron
- Component of hundreds of enzymes
- Needed for synthesis of hemoglobin
- Assists antioxidant enzymes
- Required for synthesis of DNA, amino acids, collagen, neurotransmitters, and certain hormones
- Critical for normal immune function

Beef, fortified cereal, beans, oysters, molasses, lentils, firm tofu, kidney beans, cashews, spinach, potatoes (with skin), shrimp, light tuna, eggs, tomatoes, dark meat chicken and turkey, raisins, prunes

Magnesium
- Structural component of bones
- Assists in hundreds of enzyme reactions involved in the synthesis of DNA and proteins
- Required for proper nerve conduction and muscle contraction

Pumpkin seeds, almonds, cashews, beans, spinach, milk, figs, brown rice, cocoa powder, molasses, peanuts, pineapple, okra, milk, bananas

Manganese
- Component of antioxidant enzymes
- Facilitates bone development
- Helps make and break down glucose and proteins

Brown rice, oatmeal, spinach, pineapples, almonds, pecans, molasses, whole-wheat bread, sesame seeds, peanuts, beans, sweet potatoes, tea

Molybdenum
- Assists in the metabolism of proteins, DNA, medicines, and toxins

Beans, lentils, peas, grain, nuts

Micronutrient & Function	Common Dietary Sources
MINERALS	
Phosphorus • Structural component of bones and teeth • Structural component of DNA • Structural component of cell membranes • Assists in energy production and storage	Milk, yogurt, salmon, halibut, lentils, beef, peanuts, sunflower seeds, beans, chicken, turkey, almonds, cheese, eggs, whole-wheat bread
Potassium • Maintains fluid and electrolyte balance • Required for proper nerve conduction and muscle contraction • Lowers blood pressure	Beans, potatoes (with skin), prunes, raisins, acorn squash, bananas, spinach, tomato juice, artichokes, molasses, tomatoes, oranges
Selenium • Component of antioxidant enzymes • Influences thyroid hormone function	Brazil nuts (from selenium-rich soil)*, crab meat, salmon, halibut, pasta, pork, shrimp, whole-wheat bread, brown rice, beef, light-meat chicken, milk, black walnuts *A single nut may exceed selenium recommendations.
Sodium • Maintains fluid and electrolyte balance • Required for proper nerve conduction and muscle contraction • Increases blood pressure	Baked goods, processed meat, restaurant food, pizza, canned soups, table salt Most Americans consume too much sodium. The tolerable upper intake level for sodium is 2,300 mg, the amount found in one teaspoon of table salt.

Micronutrient & Function	Common Dietary Sources
MINERALS	
Zinc • Assists in hundreds of enzyme reactions • Assists in hemoglobin production • Assists antioxidant enzymes • Supports immune function	Oysters, beef, crab meat, dark-meat chicken and turkey, pork, yogurt, milk, cashews, chickpeas, almonds, peanuts, cheese

39

How do you know what you are eating? Any food in a package will have a label that tells you the nutritional value of the food. Understanding a food label will help you identify the quantity (in grams or micrograms) of the macronutrients (fats, carbohydrates, protein), vitamins, and minerals in the foods you eat.

---

39 Table created from list Accessed March 6, 2020. https://lpi.oregonstate.edu/sites/lpi.oregonstate.edu/files/pdf/mic/micronutrients_for_health.pdf

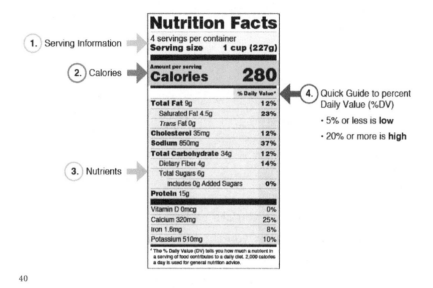

1. Serving Information

2. Calories

3. Nutrients

Nutrition Facts

4 servings per container
Serving size   **1 cup (227g)**

Amount per serving
Calories   **280**

	% Daily Value*
Total Fat 9g	**12%**
Saturated Fat 4.5g	**23%**
Trans Fat 0g	
Cholesterol 35mg	**12%**
Sodium 850mg	**37%**
Total Carbohydrate 34g	**12%**
Dietary Fiber 4g	**14%**
Total Sugars 6g	
Includes 0g Added Sugars	**0%**
Protein 15g	
Vitamin D 0mcg	0%
Calcium 320mg	25%
Iron 1.6mg	8%
Potassium 510mg	10%

* The % Daily Value (DV) tells you how much a nutrient in a serving of food contributes to a daily diet. 2,000 calories a day is used for general nutrition advice.

4. Quick Guide to percent Daily Value (%DV)

· 5% or less is **low**

· 20% or more is **high**

40

In general, adult intake of calories should come from 45-65% carbohydrates, 20-35% fat, and 10-35% protein.[41] [42] Appropriate nutritional intake is essential for recovery and repair from surgery.

40 FDA.gov https://www.fda.gov/food/nutrition-education-resources-materials/ how-understand-and-use-nutrition-facts-label

41 The National Academies of Sciences Engineering Medicine, 2002. "Dietary Reference Intakes for Energy, Carbohydrate, Fiber, Fat, Fatty Acids, Cholesterol, Protein, and Amino Acids." Accessed February 29, 2020. http://www.nationalacademies.org/hmd/ Reports/2002/Dietary-Reference-Intakes-for-Energy-Carbohydrate-Fiber-Fat-Fatty-Acids-Cholesterol-Protein-and-Amino-Acids.aspx

42 Dietary Guidelines for Americans 2015-2020, 8th edition. Accessed February 29, 2020. https://health.gov/sites/default/files/2019-09/2015-2020_Dietary_Guidelines.pdf

OPTIMIZING NUTRITION STATUS
FOR A SUCCESSFUL SURGERY

The prospect of surgery can seem daunting to anyone. The good news is you can perform simple steps before surgery to set yourself up for a better surgical outcome. Specifically, getting enough of the right kind of nourishment before and after surgery helps prevent complications. Research shows that malnutrition is very common among certain groups of patients before surgery. As many as 50% of patients enter surgery malnourished while proper nutrition is often overlooked among many of the other concerns before surgery.

It should come as no surprise that a well-nourished body is better equipped to tackle the challenge of surgery. Any surgical procedure can take its toll on the body. The operation itself leads to inflammation and metabolic stress. Patients with poor nutritional reserves can be unable to manage the demands of surgery and to activate the recovery process. If nutritional reserves are already low or at zero, and there is poor eating after surgery, the body may start breaking down existing muscle and tissue for energy and to support the healing process.

Malnutrition occurs when the body does not get the nutrients it needs and can be found in people of every size and age. Malnutrition before surgery is associated with longer hospital stays and longer recovery periods. Americans are malnourished, according to Mike Fenster, M.D., an interventional cardiologist, chef, and author of *The Fallacy of the Calorie: Why the Modern Western Diet is Killing Us and How to Stop It.* According to Fenster, the modern Western diet is replacing fresh fruits and vegetables with refined carbohydrates and other processed offerings. Not a good diet for anyone, let alone someone anticipating TKR.

There is growing evidence that good nutrition can positively affect both the quality of healing and the time needed for healing. Fortunately, some healthcare providers recognize this and provide protocols to help assess, recognize, treat, and prevent malnutrition in surgical patients. It is incumbent upon patients and healthcare providers to advocate for such protocols and to seek a holistic approach to the surgical process and the nutrition that surrounds it. Some simple suggestions include:

- Avoid long periods of fasting before surgery (except what is required by your doctor immediately prior to surgery).
- Start oral feeding as soon as possible after surgery.
- Start nutrition therapy early (pre-operatively) or as soon as nutritional risk becomes apparent.
- As soon as you know you are having surgery, ask for a blood test for general screening with additional panels for iron, vitamins, and minerals. After consulting with your health care professional, consider making adjustments to your diet or supplementation to address any deficiencies.

Sample post-operative vitamins/supplements:

Vitamin K
- Promotes clotting to help heal incisions after surgery
- Builds strong bones (healing around your implant)
- Found in green leafy vegetables

Grape Seed Extract

- Enhances wound healing
- Promotes healthy blood vessels
- Reduces swelling after surgery
- Taken in capsule/tablet form

Coenzyme Q10

- Speeds metabolism—healing of tissues
- Reduces pain
- Helps control bleeding
- Taken in capsules/tablets

Arnica

- Stimulates circulation
- Reduce inflammation and pain
- Taken in tablets dissolved under the tongue
- Can be applied topically once the incision has healed

Fish Oils

- Anti-inflammatory
- Strengthen the heart's electrical system
- Found in cold-water fish such as salmon, trout, mackerel, and tuna

Turmeric and Curcumin

- Anti-inflammatory
- Antioxidant—protects the body from free radicals that can harm the body
- Take in liquid form for best results, as absorption starts in the mouth

GETTING PREPARED FOR SURGERY TAKES A LITTLE PLANNING

Preparing yourself for surgery is like preparing for a procedure that creates some stress on your body. Consider pre-surgical nutrition similar to getting ready for a marathon or big game.

Pre-op Nutrition Considerations

Your pre-surgery diet should include as many nutrients as possible to improve the health of your body. At least two weeks before surgery, make sure you eat enough protein daily. The guidelines outlined earlier in the chapter provide a framework for the amount of protein necessary on a daily basis. Typically, 1.8-2.0g/kg (0.8-0.9 g/lb) per day provides optimum health. Not all protein is created equally. Most animal sources (fish, eggs, dairy, meat) deliver all the amino acids your body needs. Plant-based proteins (grains, beans, vegetables, nuts) often lack one or more of the essential amino acids but can be combined to create the complete protein.

Protein provides building blocks for muscles and bones and strengthens the immune system. Remember, you want to be as strong as possible going into surgery.

Stock up on fruits and vegetables. Include fruit and vegetables at most meals and snacks. Most specifically, ensure you include greens. Greens are great for your skin and repair muscles, bones, and cartilage. They contain loads of vitamins and minerals, including vitamins C and K and magnesium.

Include whole grains to give your body the B vitamins it needs to combat stress.

Consider reducing or eliminating additional sugars, caffeine, and alcohol from your diet. These create more stress on the body and actually remove nutrients to metabolize properly.

Post-op Nutrition Considerations

Post-op nutritional goals make it possible for a speedier recovery and help you return to doing the things you love as soon as possible. Eat smaller meals more often for optimal absorption and consistency of nutrients to facilitate healing and recovery.

Include enough fiber. Add fiber at each meal and snack, from fruits and vegetables to cooked beans and whole grains. Fiber helps maintain normal bowel movement, which will be disrupted from surgery, anesthesia, and medications. Initiate this process sooner rather than later to avoid discomfort. The top three sources in each food group are listed below:

HIGH FIBER FOODS[43]

FRUITS	Serving Size	Total Fiber (g)
Raspberries	1 cup	8.0
Pear	1 medium	5.5
Apple with Skin	1 medium	4.5
VEGETABLES	Serving Size	Total Fiber (g)
Green Peas	1 cup	9.0
Broccoli	1 cup chopped	5.0
Turnip Greens	1 cup	5.0

---

43 Mayo Clinic. "Chart of High Fiber Foods." Accessed February 29, 2020. https://www.mayoclinic.org/healthy-lifestyle/nutrition-and-healthy-eating/in-depth/high-fiber-foods/art-20050948

GRAINS	Serving Size	Total Fiber (g)
Spaghetti, whole wheat	1 cup	6.0
Barley, pearled, cooked	1 cup	6.0
Bran flakes	¾ cup	6.0
LEGUMES, SEEDS, & NUTS	**Serving Size**	**Total Fiber (g)**
Split peas	1 cup	16.0
Lentils	1 cup	15.5
Black beans	1 cup	15.0

Protein, once again, is essential. Have protein at each meal for your muscles and bones. It is found in meat, fish, eggs, poultry, nuts, dairy products, soy products, and cooked dried beans.

Calcium is important for bone healing and overall health. Drink milk or calcium-fortified juices, and eat yogurt or cheese. Your physician may recommend a calcium pill and vitamin D if you don't get enough from food or have tested positive for bone deficiency.

Wound healing is facilitated with vitamin C, which also helps form bone. Get vitamin C from citrus fruits, green and red peppers, collard greens, broccoli, spinach, strawberries, tomatoes, and potatoes.

To avoid constipation, drink at least six to eight cups of fluids each day. Better yet, consume half your body weight in ounces of water. So, if you weigh 200 pounds, drink 100 oz of water per day.

Side Note: Before we start talking about how much water to drink, we encourage you to drink water out of a reusable, refillable container. If you must purchase a disposable single-use water bottle, please recycle it.

That's five 20 oz. (reusable) water bottles, which may sound like a lot. If your body is not used to so much water, you will have to urinate more frequently as your body adjusts. With time, you will not need to use the loo so frequently, and your body will work more like a juicy orange than beef jerky. Keep a water bottle in convenient places: at your desk, in your kitchen, in your car (but keep it out of the sun), by your favorite chair, on your bedside table. Get used to taking drinks of water throughout the day. Staying adequately hydrated is often overlooked, yet one of the very best and simplest things you can do to enhance your body's function.

What Does Water Do For You?

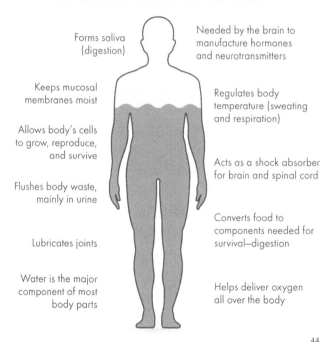

Forms saliva (digestion)

Needed by the brain to manufacture hormones and neurotransmitters

Keeps mucosal membranes moist

Allows body's cells to grow, reproduce, and survive

Flushes body waste, mainly in urine

Lubricates joints

Water is the major component of most body parts

Regulates body temperature (sweating and respiration)

Acts as a shock absorber for brain and spinal cord

Converts food to components needed for survival—digestion

Helps deliver oxygen all over the body

44

44 USGS image public domain. Accessed March 1, 2020. https://www.usgs.gov/media/images/water-you-what-water-does-your-body

Hydration is critical for recovery, healing, and general health. Drinking enough water each day is crucial to regulate body temperature, keep joints lubricated, prevent infections, deliver nutrients to cells, and keep organs functioning properly. Being well hydrated also improves sleep quality, cognition, and mood.

What exactly does hydration do for you after surgery, and how do you know if you are adequately hydrated? Let's explore the body's need for water.

Up to 60% of the human adult body is water.[45] Your blood is made up of plasma (mostly water with proteins, ions, nutrients, and wastes), red blood cells that carry oxygen and carbon dioxide, platelets (responsible for blood clotting), and white blood cells (immune response). Your blood helps to initiate and perpetuate the healing process. When tissues are dehydrated and blood volume is low, the blood becomes thicker. When the blood gets thicker, it is harder to move and starts to form clots.

One of the dreaded postoperative complications is the formation of a clot in the major veins of the legs, called deep vein thrombosis. The clot can cause extreme pain and swelling and may dislodge, traveling to the lungs and causing a pulmonary embolism. Hydration plays a vital role in preventing blood clots from forming. There is plenty of evidence showing that adequate post-operative hydration is essential in the prevention of clots.

---

45 USGS. "The Water in You: Water and the Human Body." Accessed March 6, 2020. https://www.usgs.gov/special-topic/water-science-school/science/water-you-water-and-human-body?qt-science_center_objects=0#qt-science_center_objects

During and after surgery, water is pulled from the vessels to the surgical site to initiate healing. This is the body's natural protective mechanism to fight infection and facilitate healing. Postoperative swelling is also part of the healing process taking place. You need to replenish this water as it is crucial for wound healing.

Being hydrated can decrease your postoperative pain and the need for pain medications. Remember, better hydration means more blood volume, which translates to better oxygenation of the healing tissues. That, in turn, reduces pain, helps prevent clots, and reduces constipation.

Remember, you most likely stopped eating and drinking pre-operatively and had IV fluids during and after surgery. This deprivation shuts down your intestines. Drinking fluids promotes gut motility and better absorption. Water infused with lemons and limes facilitates motility, along with other nutritional and health benefits.

Symptoms of Dehydration Include:
- Dry mouth
- Dizziness
- Lack of sweating
- Fast heart rate
- Muscle cramps
- Nausea or vomiting

By the time you get home from the hospital or same-day surgical center, you most likely have had little to drink. Your priority upon getting home is to drink and hydrate. Not only will this rehydrate your system, but it will also rid your system of toxins and anesthetics.

Monitor your progress. Your urine should be frequent and light straw in color. The darker and smellier the urine, the more dehydrated you are. If you go more than four hours without going to the bathroom, you need to increase hydration.

Keep in Mind:
- Drink lots of water infused with lemon or lime
- Stay hydrated before and after surgery
- Evaluate your hydration by monitoring your urine color.

Additional References Dr. Black Recommends:
- Centers for Disease Control and Prevention, 2020. Accessed March 1, 2020. https://www.cdc.gov/nccdphp/dnpao/data-trends-maps/index.html.
- Noakes, T, Sboros, M., 2017. *Lore of Nutrition: Challenging Conventional Beliefs*. South Africa: Penguin Books.
- Rouse, J, Rouse, D., 2014. *Think Eat Move Thrive*. New York: Simon and Schuster.
- Sumbal, M. Essential sports nutrition; a guide to optimal performance for every active person. Rockbridge Press, Emeryville, CA, 2018.

PILLAR #5 RIGHT MIND: CONSISTENCY AND POSITIVE ATTITUDE

I've included this pillar because your attitude matters. How you talk to your self and pep yourself up or put yourself down matters. I want you to know and believe that what you do, what you eat, how you prepare for surgery, and how you continue your recovery matters. We want your knee to last you many, many years and take you many places, from the blissfully pain-free mundane tasks of everyday life to grand adventures.

A theme of one of my mentors, Todd Durkin, is to "get your mind right." What he means by that is to quit the negative, degrading thoughts ("stinking thinking") and look toward the positive. He taught me about setting your own operating standards and using this as a framework to guide your life. Having your own principles and knowing your direction makes it way easier to say "Yes" and "No" at the right times.

My husband calls me the "posi-twist" because I've always had a knack for taking an unfortunate situation and finding the good. My knees are a perfect case of this. I could wallow in self-pity about having knees that forced me to pull away from so many sports and activities I loved. Instead, I choose to look at it like this: my knee condition has opened the world of cycling and prompted my quest to help you with your knees. I believe I was given these knees for that reason. In a way, I'm thankful for my wretched knees!

The two keys to the posi-twist are positive mental attitude and action on your priorities.

Many of us talk about our priorities but never take action. Let's dive a little deeper here about what role core values have in setting priorities.

Do you have your own set of guiding principles? I bet you do even though you may never have thought of it that way before. What is important to you? We each have ideas or principles that are fundamental beliefs that each of us holds as part of who we are. Values like acceptance, balance, candor, determination, empathy, freedom, gratefulness, health, integrity, joy, kindness, leadership, motivation, neatness, optimism, passion, responsibility, self-reliance, trustworthiness, understanding, vision, wonder. If you search "core values" on the web, you will find lists of hundreds of core values. It's a fun exercise to take the list and try to boil it down to no more than five core values for yourself.

I present this list to you because I hope that one particular value is on your list: health. Without your good health, nothing else matters. But it's more than just saying health is your priority; you must act on it.

If you are facing a total knee replacement, now is the time to commit to doing everything you can to make the outcome of the surgery the best it can be. This includes not just your physical actions, but your emotional energy as well. Believe that what you do to prepare will make a difference, because it will. And you need a belief the surgery will improve your life, too.

Having a positive mental attitude going into your surgery preparation, the surgery, and the recovery is key. Think about how you talk to yourself. Do you berate yourself? Are the things you say in your head anything you would say to a friend? Do you sound like your own best cheerleader, or do you have a negative soundtrack running in your head about all the things you've done wrong? If it's negative, instead try to encourage yourself. If you hear yourself nagging, just stop and think, "You can do this."

The truth is the only person who can help you is you. The only person who can change you is you. Take responsibility. Deal with your problems. Make some good choices and act on them.

> *"You are better than you think you are and*
> *can do more than you think you can."*
> —KEN CHOUBLER, FOUNDER OF THE
> LEADVILLE 100 RACE SERIES

This is my favorite quote. You can substitute the word "better" with "stronger," "smarter," "more resilient," "more persistent," and so on to give yourself some uplifting motivation.

What you say to yourself determines where you go. We all want the best outcome for you and your knees, so start visualizing that now! Think about a year from now. What is the best outcome you can imagine? See yourself smiling and enjoying life with your new knee. What are you doing? Who are you with? Where are you? Maybe you are finally taking that trip to (name the place you've always wanted to go) and can walk with ease, keep up with your family and friends, and truly enjoy the experience. Or you're on a bike ride with your friends and are leading the pack. Or maybe playing with your grandchildren, able to get off the floor grace-fully because you are so strong. Or maybe just getting in and out of the car with ease. Take just a minute and imagine your story, no matter how big or how small.

Now, work that story backward. What needs to happen for that to be true? First, prepare mentally and physically for your surgery so you are as strong as you can be going in and work your way through the recovery. Then, at about three to six months (after physical therapy), resume your training so you can do the things you hope to do. Be relentless in your commitment. Don't let things get in the way.

Sometimes you may have a setback. Real life happens. The important thing is not to let it totally derail you. Get back on track and keep moving forward.

Here's my big plan and setback story.

> I had my most recent knee replacement in November 2019. I planned the surgery in November so I would have enough time to recuperate and then train for a big bike trip in the summer. Every summer, my husband and I ride a three to four-week section while carrying our own gear, with the goal of one day completing a diagonal route from Bellingham, Washington (northwest corner) to Key West, Florida (southeast corner). My husband and I had hoped to continue with leg #3 of our bike ride across America, starting in Iowa, then heading down south along the Mississippi River. You have to be really strong to pedal and navigate because your bike plus all the gear on it weighs about 75 pounds. I'd barely have enough time to recover and train if everything went well.

At about three months post-op, I started feeling like I was done with the main part of recovery and could start slowly ramping up my weight training and increase my efforts while riding a bike. Then something very unexpected happened: my small Baker's cyst at the back of my recent TKR knee burst. Number one, I didn't know they could burst. Number two, WOW did that ever hurt! It presents like it could be a blood clot or DVT (deep vein thrombosis). My visit to the emergency room luckily confirmed that it was not a clot and "just" a burst Baker's Cyst. The fluid from the cyst (synovial fluid) causes swelling in the lower leg until it is reabsorbed over several weeks.

In the meantime, my calf felt like cement. It was so painful that I couldn't even walk and was back on crutches for a few days. It is now six weeks since that happened, and I still have pain at the back of my knee and some swelling. It totally backtracked my recovery, and I've had to take it easy, ice and elevate, and start slowly again. I'm back to really listening to my knee and not pushing the limits of pain. I continue to massage and stretch my leg, and I'm not giving up. I will reset my training plan to take into account where I am now and move ahead as my knee allows. What does this mean for our trip this summer? I don't know yet. You can check the HealthyKneesCoach.com/blog to find out what happens! If we don't make the trip in the summer of 2020, we will plan to do so in 2021. Failure is not an option because this cross-country journey is my dream and trip of a lifetime.

My point in telling you this story is that you, too, may encounter setbacks. Yes, they will be disappointing and disheartening. But don't give up! Keep your mind right, modify your plan, and keep going.

I know not everyone thinks riding a bicycle across the country is a bucket list wish come true. But what is your wish? What do you want to be able to do? Write it down and then ask yourself "what needs to be true" to make it happen. Then work your way backward, continue asking that question and writing the answers. Before you know it, you'll have a plan to reach your dream.

CHAPTER 8

TO SUM IT UP—WHERE TO GO FROM HERE

I hope the information in this book has provided solid guidance for you and your knees. If you haven't yet decided to replace your knee, I encourage you to follow the 5 Pillars to do everything you can to get stronger regardless. You might just find that you feel so much better that you don't need a knee replacement just yet.

If you've already committed to your TKR surgery, then get crackin' on the 5 Pillars! Doing some of it is better than doing none of it. I want you to be able to move ahead to surgery with confidence!

If you are post-surgery, congratulations! Do your physical therapy, and then continue on with the 5 Pillar plan. Even if your TKR was some time ago, you can still follow the plan and get great results. Sometimes clients have come to me even years after their surgeries saying their knee replacements don't feel so great. After following the plan, they are much happier. So, it is never too late! The point is that the 5 Pillar plan will help your knees no matter what.

We went over the 5 Pillar Plan in detail through the previous chapter, and we'll sum it up right here:

- Get Stronger—do exercises for your whole lower-body chain to improve muscle strength, balance, and stability.
- Move More—move your knee with cycling to improve synovial fluid production, ease discomfort, and work the range of motion without impact
- Get Flexible—improve flexibility to help your muscles and joints range of motion.
- Eat Smarter—nutritionally prepare for and recover from surgery and perhaps lose weight before surgery if that is recommended.
- Right Mind—maintain a positive mental attitude to help you through this whole process.

Here's the real scoop: TKR recovery is exhausting, especially the first two weeks, but it will be so worth it when you take that first step sometime during your recovery and experience no pain. For me, that was a feeling I never even dared to dream because I did not think it could ever be true. Yet it was, and I hope I have set you up to experience this too.

Your emotions may climb as you get a glimpse of being able to do more and crash as you hit plateaus, go backwards, or develop complications. You might even cry because of your pain and frustrations. This is where that positive mental attitude is so important. You're going to have to dig deep and find grit and power to persist.

The goal in the end is to be better off than when you started. The great news is that with the additional training recommended in this book, you can become stronger and able to move more freely than you ever thought you could.

ADDITIONAL RESOURCES

www.healthykneescoach.com/shop
www.heatlhykneescoach.com/HKstrength
www.healthykneesformula.com
Also by Robin Robertson
Book: *Healthy Knees Cycling* (2015)
Book: *Healthy & Fit Body* (2015)
Book: *Healthy Knees Strength* (2020)

THANK YOU

Thank you so much for your time in reading this book. I hope that you've learned a thing or two that will help you on your journey with your knees.

If you have any friends who suffer from knee pain, please pass this book along to them! They don't have to be facing surgery to get benefit from what we've suggested in this book. These are guidelines to help any knees feel stronger and free!

I'd love to hear your feedback! You can send me your thoughts at hello@healthykneescoach.com. If you purchased this book on Amazon, I'd sincerely appreciate a review. Reviews are so helpful to other readers that may be wondering if this book can help them too.

To your Healthy and Happy Knees,

Robin Robertson

robin@healthykneescoach.com
Facebook: healthykneescoach
www.healthykneescoach.com
www.betrainingtennis.com

ROBIN ROBERTSON

Business Owner, Founder, Author

Since 2000, Robin Robertson and her husband Doug have owned and managed the Bellingham Training and Tennis Club in Bellingham, Washington. Robin is accomplished in a variety of training methods, including Functional Aging Specialist, ACE certified personal trainer, USA Cycling Coach, author, and founder of Healthy Knees Coach.

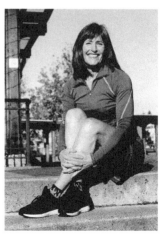

Robin is a lifelong athlete who has had a total of 12 knee surgeries. She ran competitively in high school and college but turned to cycling to save her knees. Not daunted by poor knees, in 1990, Robin and her husband toured the world on their bikes and continue on bicycle adventures every year. At age 47, Robin discovered bike racing, and in the next couple of years, placed

1st in Washington State "Best All-Around Road Rider" Masters B Division. She also raced mountain bikes, competing in the Leadville 100, among other events. She continues to train for cycling events, fitness, and multi-day self-supported bicycle adventure tours. She commutes to work and rides her bike just for fun and to keep her knees in good health. When she's not on her bike, Robin loves family time with her husband and two children and traveling to explore this amazing world. Her passion is to help others have healthy and happy knees so they too can go on many adventures.

Find Robin at
robin@healthykneescoach.com
Facebook: healthykneescoach
www.healthykneescoach.com

STEPHEN A. BLACK

DSc, M.Ed., PT, ATC/L, CSCS

Stephen A. Black is the CEO and owner of Rocky Mountain Human Performance Center (RMHPC) with offices in Boulder, Colorado, and Fort Myers, Florida. Stephen has 40+ years' experience in the health and wellness industry. He has traveled the globe promoting healthy lifestyles and providing expert insight and research in areas related to rehabilitation, fitness, and sports specific training. He has worked with professional teams, including NFL, NBA, NHL, WNBA, and ABL/NBL affiliates.

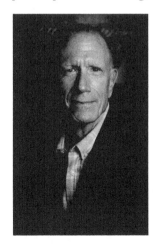

Stephen is an Associate Professor in the College of Health Professions at Florida Gulf Coast University in Fort Myers, Florida. Dr. Black's academic responsibilities include didactic and laboratory courses in anatomy, physiology, biomechanics, and cardiac pathology. His research pursuits are in the areas of endurance cardiac medicine and optimization of functional movement strategies.

As a Physical Therapist, Athletic Trainer and Strength and Conditioning Coach, Stephen utilizes his expertise and experience to the benefit of his clients. Currently, Stephen oversees clinical and research operations at RMHPC, an exercise testing, and prescription facility. RMHPC provides individualized programs for athletes, weekend warriors, and post-rehab clients. In addition to his responsibilities mentioned above, Stephen is a much sought after and respected lecturer, author, and consultant to the health and wellness industry. He serves as an advisor to several organizations and non-profit entities.

In his spare time, Stephen enjoys recreational activities such as running, cycling, swimming, skiing, and experiential activities that lead to a balanced/integrated lifestyle. He has completed multiple endurance events, including the Ironman World Championship in Kona, Hawaii. Stephen's passion is in assisting others to achieve the lifestyle they aspire to.

Rocky Mountain Human Performance Center, Inc.
www.rockymoutainhpc.com
7331 College PKWY Suite 220, Fort Meyers, FL 33907

HEALTHYKNEESFORMULA.COM

We know you might be worried about doing things the right way, and that's why we created the Healthy Knees Formula for you.

This online program will help guide you every step of the way with a week by week coached program, so you know you are doing the right thing at the right time.

We know this isn't for everyone, because to get the results, you have to do the work. We've had hundreds of clients over the past five years of running this program who have successfully reduced or eliminated their knee pain and are back to living the life they love. We think you should have this chance too.

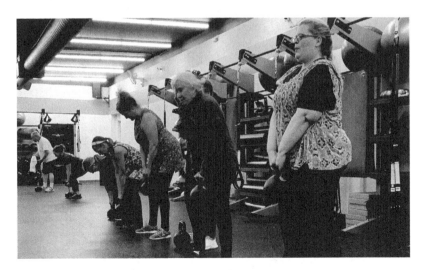

OUR FULL HEALTHY KNEES FORMULA PROGRAM INCLUDES:

Stage 1: Knee Resolve—Starting where you are with a strength-building program to stabilize your knee and stop the downward spiral.

Stage 2: Knee Relief—Reduce pain through strength training + cycling foundation to build your base.

Stage 3: Knee Rebuilding—Build strength through muscular development + cycling for knee mobility and stamina.

Stage 4: Knee Restore—Become powerful with a sense of knee freedom through a higher level of cycling and strength training.

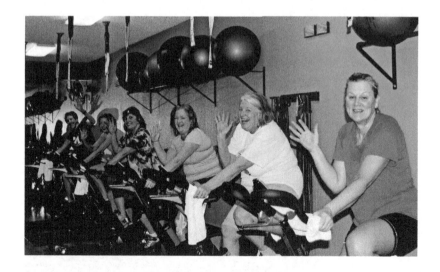

Excited to get started?
Visit us at healthykneesformula.com

Made in the USA
Columbia, SC
03 September 2020